YOUR CHILD'S BEST FACE

HOW TO **NURTURE** **TOP HEALTH** & **NATURAL GLOW**

DR. FELIX LIAO, DDS

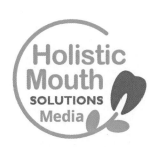

Holistic
Mouth
SOLUTIONS
Media

YOUR CHILD'S BEST FACE
HOW TO **NURTURE TOP HEALTH** & **NATURAL GLOW**

For excerpts permission, contact info@HolisticMouthSolutions.com

V1.0
ISBN: 979-8-9864268-1-5 (E)
ISBN: 979-8-9864268-0-8 (P)

Cover Design by **Rupa Limbu**

Published by **Holistic Mouth Solutions Media**

Printed in **The United States of America**

Holistic Mouth Solutions Media
7115 Leesburg Pike, Ste 310
Falls Church, VA 22043
800-969-8035
www.HolisticMouthSolutions.com

Disclaimer
The opinions, advice and recommendations in this book are intended for a wide audience of people and are not tailored or specific to individual needs or health conditions. This book is not intended as a substitute for professional medical or dental advice, diagnosis, or treatment. Always seek professional medical advice from your dentist, physician or other qualified healthcare provider with any questions you may have regarding a medical condition. This book is not intended to diagnose, treat, or cure any disease. Significant changes in your health regime should be discussed with your healthcare provider. The authors and publishers of this book make no warranty, representation, or guarantee regarding the advice given in this book, nor do they assume any liability whatsoever arising out of your use of any information or product referenced in this book.

CONTENTS

ENDORSEMENTS

"Our genes are not our destiny. Crowded teeth and braces need not be inevitable. Dr. Liao's insightful book shows parents how to recognize red flags early, what steps to take, and who can provide proactive guidance. Should treatment be needed, Dr. Liao's integrated WholeHealth approach gives children the best chance to thrive with nourishing sleep supported by the wide-open airway that comes with Best Face."

— Karen D. Cheng, *MD*
Board-certified in Sleep Medicine & Neurology
Laguna Hills, CA

"Dr. Liao's latest book is essential reading for parents who are looking for deeper explanations and solutions, and who want to put their children on the path of excellent health for life. Dr. Liao explains and illustrates with photos the importance of mouth and jaw health in the overall picture of wellness."

— Emily Pyenson, *Mom of 3*

"From impaired mouth to your child's best face, this book is a roadmap to giving your child their best lease on life. Dr. Liao gets straight to the point and explains the steps needed to get your child's health on track."

— Hallie Bulkin, *MA CCC-SLP, COM, QOM*
Certified Orofacial Myologist, Feeding Specialist
Bethesda, Maryland

"Dr. Liao does it again! This book is the perfect resource for parents wanting to learn proper steps for optimal oral/overall health. They will be empowered to guide their children's Best Face and top health by ensuring jaw growth and development to full genetic potential, and early detection by an airway focused dentist. As a dental hygienist and health care advocate, I will personally recommend this book to ALL parents."

— Lauren Gueits, *BS, RDH*
Founder & CEO
Airway Health Solutions

Your Child's Best Face is a must read for parents and practitioners responsible for the health of children! This mini book is packed with eye opening insights on the mouth as the start of many seemingly unrelated conditions — not only crooked teeth and teeth grinding, but also epilepsy, scoliosis, seasonable affect disorder (SAD), and failure to thrive. Dr. Felix provides easy to identify clues for parents and training opportunities for dentists and all types of practitioners, through his ground breaking Airway Mouth Doctor Training. You will never view your child or dentist the same way again after reading this book.

— Kimberly B. Whittle
Founder & CEO
KnoWEwell

ABOUT DR. FELIX LIAO

Dr. Felix Liao has put the missing mouth back on the healthcare map with his 3 Amazon bestsellers: *Six-Foot Tiger Three Foot Cage*, *Early Sirens*, and *Licensed to Thrive*.

Dr. Felix coined the ground-breaking term Impaired Mouth Syndrome in 2017 to reconnect the mouth with whole body health. This recognition has led to painless treatment with breakthroughs in chronic pain and fatigue, teeth grinding, brain fog, scoliosis, straighter teeth without braces and more, in both adults and children.

Dr. Felix's books and achievements have established him as a thought leader in healthcare innovation, and a pioneering Airway Mouth Doctor (AMD).

In addition to being the Director of AMD Training & Mentoring, Dr. Felix enjoys seeing patients 2 days a week in his Falls Church office in Virginia.

Felix came to America from Taiwan at age 16 and has been a U.S. citizen since 1971. His personal interests include classical music, living an organic lifestyle, the outdoors, hiking, swimming, dancing, science, international cuisine and culture, and making healthy food tasty.

FOREWORD
By Dr. Ben Miraglia, DDS

Co-Founder at Airway Health Solutions
Clinical Faculty at CandidPro
Board of Directors at American Academy of Physiological Medicine and Dentistry
President's Council at Northern Westchester Hospital

Your Child's Best Face by Dr. Felix Liao lays out the crucial connections between children's oral-facial development and their overall health and wellness for parents.

Here's why this matters: Today, many children struggle with and receive treatment for symptoms such as ADHD, bedwetting, night terrors, restless sleep, teeth grinding, ear infections, digestive issues, academic struggles, and behavioral issues. Having treated thousands of children over two decades, I have learned that there is a vast difference between treating the symptoms and treating the root cause. Rarely does treating the symptoms result in a healthy child.

The above symptoms, and many others, share a common root cause: poor breathing while sleeping. In adults, we call this Obstructive Sleep Apnea, but in children, it is referred to as Sleep Disordered Breathing. Nearly all children in industrialized countries exhibit underdeveloped jaws. This is why parents are seeing crowded teeth and mouth breathing in so many children. In this book, Dr. Felix Liao connects the epidemic of compromised airways in children with the symptoms I've mentioned above.

Healthy nasal breathing with effortless lip seal is only achievable through fully developed jaws that support 32 teeth in a broad wide arch and deliver a large airway to support deep sleep. Almost no child can achieve this naturally today. Fortunately, Dr. Felix Liao's pioneering work to train airway-centered mouth doctors with WholeHealth skill set well beyond drilling and filling is finally changing this.

Your Child's Best Face is every parent's opportunity to nurture their child through early jaw growth and set them on a path to being a healthy adult. You're about to learn how you as a parent can effectively champion your child's Best Face with top health and natural glow.

AUTHOR'S NOTE & ACKNOWLEDGEMENTS

Dear Parents,

We all want a good life with great health for our children. How your child's jaws develop before age 12 has a huge influence on his or her facial appearance and overall health as an adult. Deficient jaws lead to crowded and crooked teeth, lackluster look, weak chin, parted lips, long face, narrow palate, and more medical, dental, and mood troubles later in life.

It's time to widen our viewfinders to see the pivotal role of the mouth in a growing child's overall health. This short book shows you the red flags in dental-facial development: chapped lips, cranky moods, bunched-up teeth, teeth grinding, frequent cavities and respiratory infections, poor posture, head tilt, bed wetting and more, plus what to do about them.

Your Child's Best Face shows the transformation from duckling to swan with real-life cases. You will learn to nurture your child for a fuller face and straighter teeth — without drugs, surgery, needles, and in some cases even without braces. You will discover a new breed of dentists trained as Airway Mouth Doctors (AMDs) to provide professional guidance toward your child's Best Face in chapter 1.

An AMD is a dentist with additional training beyond teeth and gums in oral contributions to overall health. An AMD has an expanded skill set on oral facial growth in adults and children to help widen airway, support sleep, and align head-jaws-spine to bring on vibrant health without surgery or medications.

This book provides new awareness and possibilities, not medical or dental advice. Individualized care can only be provided by your doctor, dentist, or AMD. To keep this book short and sweet, only a fraction of the science is included. Readers seeking more in-depth information are encouraged to refer to books listed under Resources on page 94. If you find some messages are repetitive, it's done intentionally to emphasize those points.

Deep gratitude goes to all the parents who granted permission to share their children's case images and stories to advance the collective awareness on this topic, and to all my mentors who inspired me. In particular, this author gratefully acknowledges the teachings of Dr. Richard Beistle, Dr. Jay Gerber, Tom Magill, and Dr. G. Dave Singh for his pioneering research in Pneumopedics and Craniofacial Epigenetics.

Great appreciation goes to all the Airway Mouth Doctors: dentists who have undergone the necessary training to diagnose and treat Impaired Mouth Syndrome in their community.

Heartfelt thanks go to Dr. David Gruder for his brilliant coaching, Denise Neumann as AMD Training Coordinator and my multi-talented right hand, Aron Plucinski as video producer & director, Jessie Martin as office manager, Chef Franklin for providing *Cook2Thrive* to AMDs and their patients, Cara Duty and Brooke Goode my editors, Kimberly Whittle my Guide, BK Suru for expert formatting, Julie Chen for wonderful home cooking and writing space.

For best results, I suggest you read this book in the order presented, including taking your own Impaired Mouth Syndrome self-survey next.

Raising a child can be quite challenging at times. Nurturing Best Face for top health can be a great joy. I hope this book helps you.

Felix Liao, DDS
Falls Church, Virginia USA
October 2022

IMPAIRED MOUTH SYNDROME SCORE
A Self-Survey for Parents & Children

Impaired Mouth Syndrome is a vast set of common medical, dental, mental, and mood symptoms stemming from impaired mouth structure such as undersized jaws, crowded teeth, oversized tongue, tongue-tie, etc. These symptoms can be aggravated by impaired Mouth Style, as in consuming food and drinks that promote inflammation, obesity, and degeneration.

To determine if you, as a parent, have Impaired Mouth Syndrome, simply fill out this self-survey with the blue heading. Doing this will help you better see the red flags on your child's face and mouth.

Impaired Mouth Syndrome Score

by Dr. Felix Liao, DDS, Author of *Six-foot Tiger, Three-foot Cage*

Mouth	Score	Body	Score
Snoring, morning dry mouth	0 1	Gasping or choking in sleep	0 1
Teeth grinding, jaw clenching	0 1	Neck, shoulder, or back pain; headaches	0 1
Mouth breathing, chapped lips	0 1	Erectile dysfunction or PMS	0 1
Persistent/wandering dental sensitivity	0 1	High blood pressure, heart disease	0 1
Gum recession and/or redness	0 1	Diabetes type 2, bloating after meals	0 1
Clicking/locking jaw joints, zigzag jaw opening	0 1	Weight gain, pot belly; acid reflux	0 1
Morning headache and/or sore jaws	0 1	Daytime sleepiness, fatigue	0 1
Deep overbite or underbite (weak chin)	0 1	Senile memory, ADD/ADHD	0 1
Frequent cavities or broken/chipped teeth	0 1	Frequent colds, flu, and skin disorders	0 1
Teeth prints on the sides of the tongue	0 1	Obstructive sleep apnea from a sleep test	0 1
Bony outgrowth on palate or inside lower jaw	0 1	Stuffy/runny nose, scratchy/itchy throat	0 1
Sunken lips and reverse smile curve (sad)	0 1	Forward head: ears ahead of shoulders	0 1
History of teeth extractions for braces	0 1	Waking up to urinate more than once	0 1
Bulge under lower jaw, double chin	0 1	Large neck size (M>17, W>15)	0 1
History of lots of dental work + medical symptoms	0 1	Poor digestion and elimination	0 1
Malocclusion (crowded teeth)	0 1	Depression, anxiety, grouchiness	0 1
Total Score		Total Score	

www.HolisticMouthSolutions.com

Figure 1

Impaired Mouth Syndrome (IMS) Score is intended as a survey of symptoms, not to indicate severity or prognosis. The combined score is not as important as the Mouth-Body connections and the resulting solutions.

Experience has shown that many symptoms, whether medical, dental, mental, or emotional, improve when impaired Mouth is correctly diagnosed and treated. This requires a dentist turned mouth doctor with an additional skill set and wider knowledge bases.

Why Does Impaired Mouth Syndrome Matter for Children?

Impaired Mouth Syndrome is missing on the radar of nearly all doctors and dentists as of 2022. Parents can take charge of their child's dental-facial development proactively starting with this survey.

Child Name: _____   Date: _____

Parent Name: _____   Contact: _____

Red Flags re: Your Child's Best Face

Mouth	Score	Body	Score
Lips chapped, peeling, or blue	0 1	Waking up tired or cannot get up	0 1
Mouth breathing (lips apart) habitually	0 1	Excessive daytime sleepiness	0 1
White shows between eye lid and pupil	0 1	Not sleeping through the night	0 1
Facial asymmetry: one eye higher, one mouth corner lower, ears uneven	0 1	Allergies, dark circle under eyes	0 1
Nostrils uneven, narrow, tiny	0 1	Stuffy/runny nose, ear tubes	0 1
Upper & lower dental midlines off	0 1	Uneven shoulders, scoliosis	0 1
Teeth grinding sounds or worn teeth	0 1	Bed wetting	0 1
Cavities-prone, red/bleeding gums	0 1	Under weight & height in growth	0 1
Swallow with gurgling sounds, bobbing head ("goose necking"), grimaced face	0 1	Obstructive sleep apnea diagnosed from sleep test	0 1
Tongue-tie, tongue thrust, tooth prints on the sides of the tongue	0 1	Slumped posture, head forward: ears ahead of shoulders	0 1
Frequent sighing or yawning	0 1	Learning or behavior problems	0 1
Thumb sucking, nail biting; narrow & high palate	0 1	Tired, listless, lethargic, cranky, depressed, anxious, moody	0 1
Weak chin, double chin	0 1	Overweight, low thyroid function	0 1
Malocclusion: crowded/crooked teeth, deep bite, open bite, cross bite, etc.	0 1	Snoring, snorting, choking in sleep	0 1
Total Score		Total Score	

www.HolisticMouthSolutions.com

Figure 2

What Is an AMD?

AMD is short for Airway Mouth Doctor. An AMD is a family dentist with additional WholeHealth training to diagnose and treat Impaired Mouth Syndrome in both kids and adults. An AMD provides:

- Early detection of red flags as shown in chapter 2.
- Referrals to like-minded experts to set the body on the right track.
- Guidance on diet and lifestyle to grow jaws and prevent teeth crowding.
- Referrals and recommendations for nasal breathing, myofunctional therapy, tongue-tie release, and healthier eating.
- Epigenetic oral appliances with desired corrections baked in.

Epi- is Greek for "on top of, or in addition to". Think of epigenetic as external assist to genes at work.

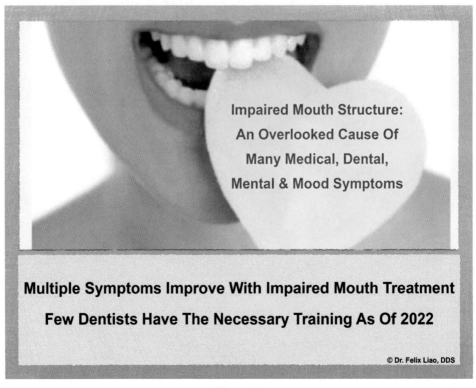

Figure 3

Proactive Benefits for Children

With the right diagnosis and treatment for Impaired Mouth Syndrome, the benefits for children can include the following within the limits of the genes inherited and parental compliance:

- Better learning and focus from better sleep.
- Less anxiety and/or depression from easier breathing.
- Wider airway from fuller jaw growth.
- Better socializing from better mood.
- Fuller jaw growth from bone-building diet.
- Less dental crowding from fuller jaws.
- Better face from fuller jaws, no tongue-tie, 100% lip seal and nasal breathing.

INTRODUCTION
Best Face Defined

We humans have an innate ability to read a face and instantly tell if it's in pain and distress or glowing with health. Just as the eyes are the windows to the soul, the face is the mirror reflecting one's physical health and emotional state.

"Best Face" in this book is defined as dental-facial development reaching full genetic potential within the genes inherited from parents. Barring genetic defects and inherited traits of facial deformity like a Hapsburg nose, full genetic potential comes with these features:

- Wide-open airway between the nose and the throat.
- Well-developed jaws for all 16 teeth to line up straight in each jaw.
- Well-coordinated "peak to valley" fit of upper/lower teeth.
- Upper and lower dental midlines aligned with the body's long axis.
- Spacious "home office" between both jaws for the tongue.
- Balanced facial features, high cheek bones, and lip seal.

Best Face is based on insights I gained from treating thousands of adult Impaired Mouth cases. Impaired Mouth is simply the deficient development of the jaws, face, and airway that is not noticed during the formative years. The result is impaired health, short of Best Face.

As various medical, dental, and mood symptoms subsided or vanished with Impaired Mouth treatment in adults, my patients were delighted. Connecting these dots led to this book for parents. With Best Face comes top health and more. It's simply the Law of Form and Function.

Imagine for a moment that you are a movie director. Which of the two faces in Figure 4 would you cast as lead actress?

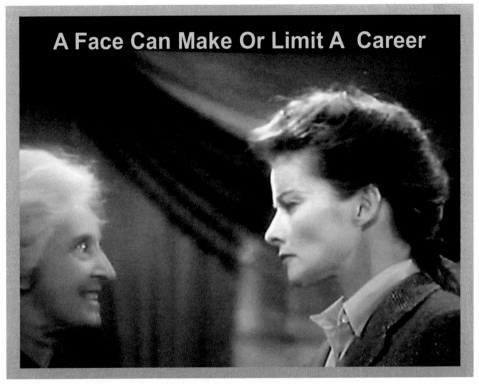

Figure 4. *Two-thirds of the human face is supported from below by the two jaws.*

In Figure 4, the face on the left failed to thrive during growth years, where-as the face on the right grew into its full genetic potential. Which face would you choose for your child?

Now look at Figure 5 and you will see that the actress on the left in Figure 4 has Liao's Sign, a surface clue for weak mid-face and narrower airway in adults that can handicap overall health.

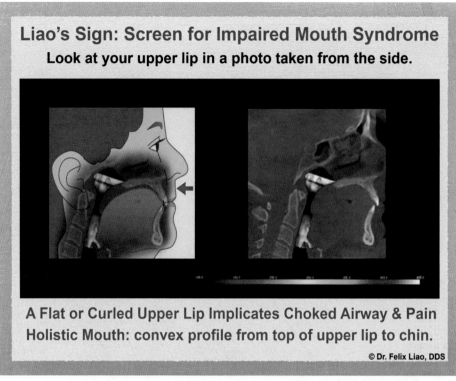

Liao's Sign: Screen for Impaired Mouth Syndrome
Look at your upper lip in a photo taken from the side.

A Flat or Curled Upper Lip Implicates Choked Airway & Pain
Holistic Mouth: convex profile from top of upper lip to chin.

© Dr. Felix Liao, DDS

Figure 5. Color scale: White means the airway is wide-open like a four-lane highway, while black means one-lane width or less. White is strong oxygen supply, while red is poor.

What's new: As a parent, you are no longer a sitting duck not knowing whether your child will end up with bunched-up teeth, closed-down airway, and half-stunted face. The pages ahead will show you how to bring on your child's Best Face with wider airway to promote jaw growth to full genetic potential with room for all 32 teeth to come in straight.

Meet Your Jaws

Maxilla is the upper jaw that supports the mid-face from the corners of the eyes to the corners of the mouth and ear to ear, as shown in purple in Figure 6. A well-formed maxilla results in higher cheek bones, fuller lips, a wider airway, higher energy, and fewer health troubles.

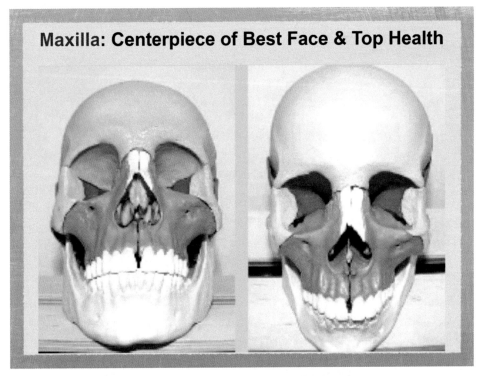

Maxilla: Centerpiece of Best Face & Top Health

Figure 6. *Maxilla is purple and mandible is white.*

A deficient maxilla has serious health consequences beyond jumbled teeth and weak mid-face. They can include sleep apnea, teeth grinding chronic pain and fatigue, and more, as shown in your own Impaired Mouth Syndrome Score on page 11.

Mandible (lower jaw) forms the lower third of your face. Over- or under-development of the mandible can lead to:

- A weak chin that is susceptible to sleep apnea and jaw pain.

- A huge chin results in a "witchy" profile.

- Double chin means no jaw line and higher risk of sleep apnea.

- Long and narrow "horsey" adult face from habitual mouth breathing with lips apart unnoticed during growing years.

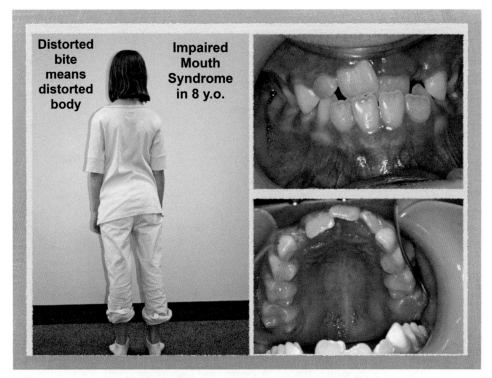

Figure 7. *Deficient jaws and crowded teeth in bad bite can twist posture in children and cause pain in adults.*

An undersized maxilla is a root cause of teeth crowding in children, as Figure 7 shows. It can also contribute to waking up tired, moodiness, ADD/ADHD, frequent respiratory infections, pediatric sleep apnea, bed wetting, and more.

Such symptoms are rooted in an Impaired Mouth with deficient jaws and choked airway. *"A syndrome is a recognizable complex of symptoms and physical findings which indicate a specific condition for which a direct cause is not necessarily understood."* as defined by <u>American Medical Information Association</u>[1].

In the case of Impaired Mouth Syndrome, the direct cause is clear based on clinical experience: a deficient maxilla that failed to grow fully for all adults teeth showing up, as in Figure 8.

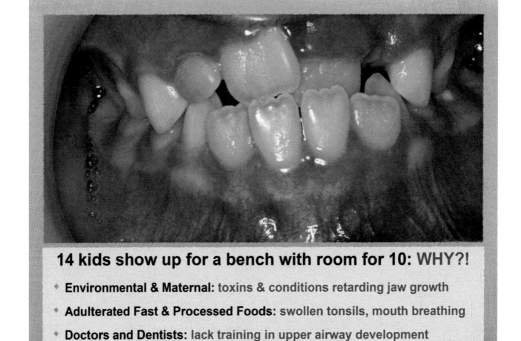

14 kids show up for a bench with room for 10: WHY?!

* **Environmental & Maternal:** toxins & conditions retarding jaw growth
* **Adulterated Fast & Processed Foods:** swollen tonsils, mouth breathing
* **Doctors and Dentists:** lack training in upper airway development

© Dr. Felix Liao, DDS

Figure 8

Underdeveloped jaws can result in pediatric obstructive sleep apnea. This most important finding is shown in Figure 9. It means:

A. Sleep apnea in adults is simply Impaired Mouth left undiagnosed from childhood on.

B. Early recognition and treatment of Impaired Mouth is the best prevention for sleep apnea and many other conditions.

C. Optimal oral-facial growth in childhood is the root-cause solution to avoid Impaired Mouth Syndrome.

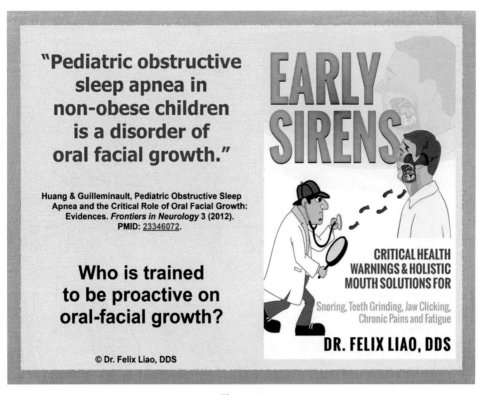

Figure 9

We were all one-year old once, like my granddaughter Camila in Figure 10, full of possibilities ahead. Will she grow up with top health and a natural glow? Will your child? That's why I wrote this book.

How to bring out my kid's best face and top health?

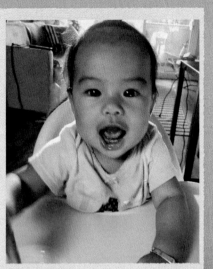

- ❖ **It's NOT any appliance!**
- ❖ **Parent-Doctor Partnership**
- ❖ **Committed Parents:**
  - ❖ **See red flags & act early**
  - ❖ **Nurture sound diet & airway**
- ❖ **Trained Mouth Doctors:**
  - ❖ **Airway-centered, not just teeth**
  - ❖ **Guide jaw & facial growth to full genetic potential**

Figure 10

As parents, we can either nurture oral-facial growth toward Best Face now or pay for the medical-dental consequences of Impaired Mouth later.

Not Knowing Has Consequences

The 10-year-old in Figures 11 and 12 came with terrible jaw deformity from habitual mouth breathing. Chronic nasal obstruction was the root cause of her long face, tongue thrust, and lip incompetence, which in turn is rooted in a deficient maxilla and standard American diet. No one ever educated her mom about what mouth breathing can do to her daughter's teeth, jaws, and face. Her dental office operated within the traditional box of fixing cavities.

Habitual mouth breathing is a serious red flag. Not knowing this can have significant dental-facial consequences. Worse yet, some treatment can aggravate Impaired Mouth Syndrome, as the chapters ahead will show.

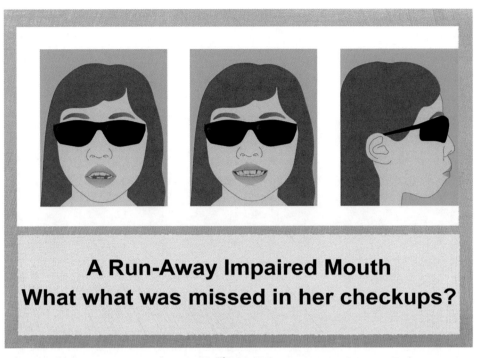

Figure 11

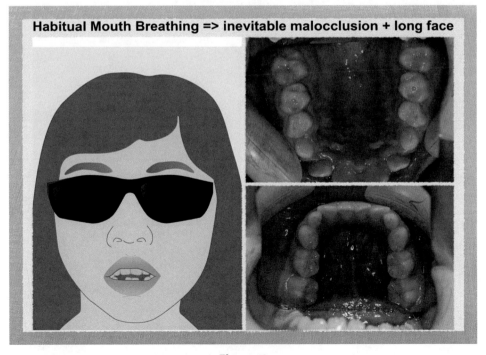

Figure 12

There's a straight and natural path to grow your child's Best Face. Staying on it is full of challenges, as in Figures 7, 8, 11, and 12. When needed, a palatal (maxilla) expander paired to a bone-building diet can be used to achieve sufficient jaw growth for all teeth to line up straight. The chapters ahead will show you the WholeHealth logic to optimize a child's growth and development, as shown in Figures 13 and 14.

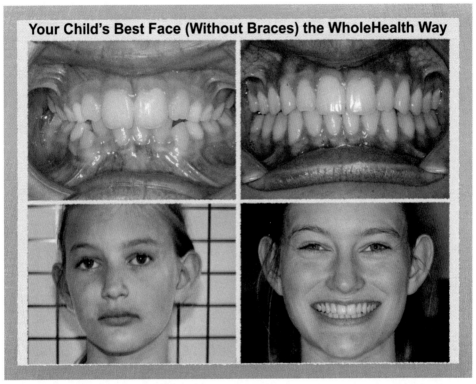

Your Child's Best Face (Without Braces) the WholeHealth Way

Figure 13. *Based on her treatment, RH is aspiring to be an Airway Mouth Doctor herself.*

What makes a face glow? First, it's the energy from a great night's sleep which is dependent on a wide airway from a well-formed maxilla. A sound diet is also important.

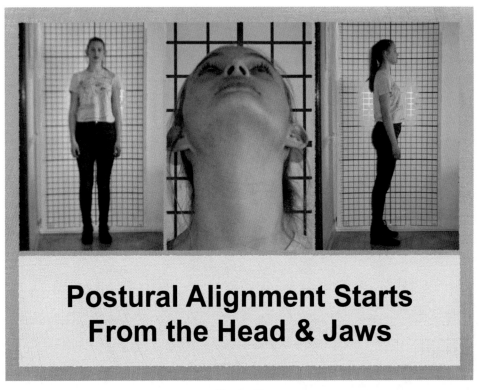

Figure 14

A fully developed maxilla is the centerpiece of Best Face and the key stone for top health in children. Now, let's see how you can bring on your child's Best Face.

CHAPTER 1
BETTER FACE, BETTER HEALTH
"Oral Health Is More Than Healthy Teeth"
David Satcher, MD, US Surgeon General

All parents want their children to be healthy, sociable, and successful in school, sports, the arts, and life. Achieving all that requires lots of energy. The mouth is the source of this energy through diet and airway. In this book, we will focus on the origin of a wide-open airway: a fully developed set of jaws in the facial skeleton.

A good face comes with much more than straight white teeth for smiles. A well-developed facial structure delivers better breathing, sleeping, eating, learning, and more room for teeth to line up straight naturally. Similarly, a flat or scrunched face means more teeth crowding, pain, fatigue, learning issues, and colds and flus.

Simply put: better face, better health.

Maxilla: Maximally Important

The human head is made of 22 bones; 14 of them frame the face, the eye sockets, nose, cheek bones, and two jaws. Maxilla is the upper jaw that props up your midface from the inside.

Maxilla is maximally important because it is the centerpiece of the face. In a fully grown maxilla, teeth align naturally from the *normal* use of the lips, cheek, and tongue.

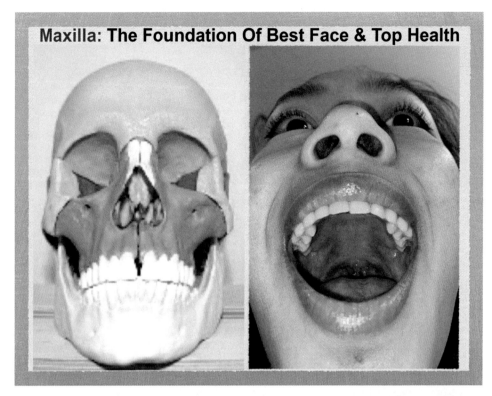

Figure 15. *A fully developed maxilla (purple bone) is the foundation for your child's Best Face. Wide space between the roof and the floor of the mouth is vital to avoid airway obstruction.*

"Normal" here means no mouth breathing from stuffy nose, no tongue-tie, and no tongue thrust in abnormal swallows 2,000 times a day — these are basic conditions for sound facial growth, as you will see ahead.

Mandible is your lower jaw. The tongue is attached to the mandible, while the jaw joints (TMJs) connect the mandible to the head just in front of the ears. Mandible adapts to and follows maxilla. Facial radiance and natural health show up when:

- Maxilla grows fully for all teeth to come in straight.
- Mandible fits into maxilla without having to go sideway or backward.
- The tongue has enough space in the mouth to stay out of the throat.

Figures 16 and 17 reinforce WHY maxilla matters to the face and the whole body.

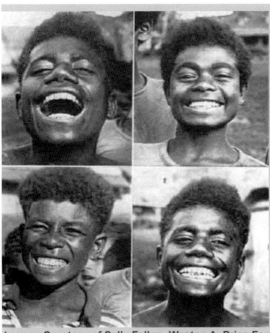

Natural Wellness

Full genetic potential looks and works like this:

- Broad **faces**
- Wide **arches**
- Balanced **head and jaws**
- **High cheekbones**
- **Radiant health**
- **Spontaneous joy**
- **No need for pediatricians**
- **No need for braces**

Images Courtesy of Sally Fallon, Weston A. Price Foundation.

Figure 16

The Teeth Tell the Tale!

STRAIGHT TEETH WIDE Dental Arches	CROOKED, CROWDED TEETH Narrow Dental Arches
Plenty of room in head for pituitary, pineal, hypothalamus	Compromised space for master glands in the head
Good skeletal development, good muscles	Poor development, poor posture, easily injured
Keen eyesight and hearing	Poor eyesight and hearing
Optimal function of all organs	Compromised function of all organs
Optimistic outlook, learns easily	Depression, behavior problems, learning problems
Round pelvic opening, easy childbirth	Oval pelvic opening, difficult childbirth

Slide Courtesy of Sally Fallon, WAP Foundation

Figure 17

A Deficient Maxilla Starts Impaired Mouth Syndrome

When a maxilla fails to thrive, the mandible is forced towards the ears and throat. Then jaw clicking and pain follow. Many medical, dental, and mood symptoms can arise from such an Impaired Mouth, including but not limited to:

- Crowded teeth, jaw clenching, teeth grinding.
- Narrower airway, less oxygen, and poor sleep.
- Persistent pain, chronic fatigue, anxiety, and depression.
- Excessive wear of teeth and jaw joints clicking/popping/locking.
- Lower energy, weaker chin, tired face, depressed look, and more.
- Higher dental and medical bills.

Living and sleeping with an Impaired Mouth is like going through life with a bad back — you don't thrive, and you don't feel your best. Raising your child toward Best Face can help avoid that fate.

Airway-Centered Mouth Doctors (AMD)

An AMD is a family dentist with additional training to diagnose and treat oral contributions to Impaired Mouth Syndrome in adults and children. Seeing an AMD involves no shots, drills, pain, drugs, or surgery except for tongue-tie and lip-tie release.

AMD is not a formal or higher degree. However, an AMD does operate from a wider WholeHealth knowledge base than teeth and gums. An AMD works with like-minded health professionals to restore whole body health. An AMD focuses on oral contributions to airway, sleep, growth, as well as systemic influence on oral health such as thyroid function and nutrition.

As an AMD, I work first as a health detective on a patient's mouth structure and usage. If either jaw is underdeveloped, I then figure out what's off and where. Based on WholeHealth assessment of the mouth and the rest of the body, I then design and use retainer-like expanders (oral appliances) as needed to grow and align the jaws, to relieve dental crowding, support sleep, widen the airway, and promote jaw growth. This oral appliance treatment is done in combination with a bone-building diet, as the cases ahead will show.

Myofunctional Therapists

An AMD works closely with myofunctional therapists. Think of them as physical therapists for all the mouth muscles: the lips, cheeks, tongue, and throat. (*Myo-* means muscle in Greek). The actions of these muscles have the power to shape the face or disfigure it, as shown in Figures 11-12 and the next case.

Snorers, mouth breathers, and tongue thrusters need myofunctional therapists' expertise and guidance on mouth-brain integration.

"The tongue is a respiratory organ. Restoring nasal breathing requires reeducation...", says Dr. Takashi Ono[2]. That's why myofunctional work is foundational to Best Face. Now let's put all these points to work.

Best Face & Top Health Starts with Seeing Impaired Mouth

HR came with a referral from her mom's chiropractors Drs. Lim & Krakos: "I need a new night guard because I've ground through the one my orthodontist gave me." She had her braces taken off four years earlier. As Figure 18 shows, her night guard failed because teeth grinding continued. Knowing the WHY behind teeth grinding is the key to a new life-changing solution.

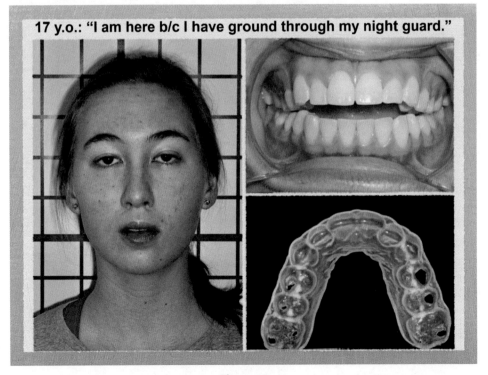

17 y.o.: "I am here b/c I have ground through my night guard."

Figure 18

The gap between HR's upper and lower front teeth is called Anterior Open Bite (AOB). The direct cause of AOB is the tongue struggling in the squeezed confine between undersized jaws. A tongue fighting to stay out of the throat (to keep the airway open) has the power to pry the front teeth apart and undo straight teeth after braces. With HR's teeth grinding came waking up tired, pain in and around her jaw joints, and not enough stamina to win tennis matches.

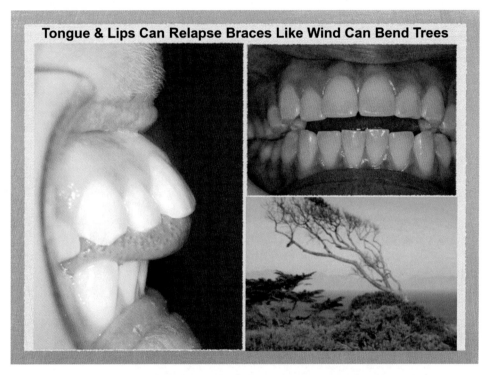

Figure 19. *Just as the wind can bend a tree, tongue thrust can pry teeth apart trying to stay out of the airway.*

After my explanation, HR and her mom chose to fix the root cause: regrow her deficient maxilla using an epigenetic oral appliance as part of a WholeHealth treatment plan.

Failure to grow maxilla sufficiently leads to Impaired Mouth Syndrome, narrower airway, and crowded teeth. Failure to diagnose Impaired Mouth Syndrome and treat its root cause can result in many medical and dental symptoms on top of relapse after braces.

In particular, Anterior Open Bite cases require WholeHealth teamwork, including but not limited to:

- An AMD to widen the home-office space for the tongue, and tongue-tie release as needed.
- A qualified myofunctional therapist to help retrain the tongue to swallow normally.
- Parental support and patient effort to achieve lip seal by unblocking the nose with necessary diet change (see chapter 4 ahead), nasal hygiene, and breathing exercise.

In addition, specialized physical therapy and chiropractics may be needed based on the full diagnosis of a trained AMD.

Figures 20–23 show the results that a night guard can never deliver. Credit goes to HR for being fully compliant with wearing her oral appliance 16 hours a day. She switched from a fast food and junk food diet favored by American teens to an organic, bone-building diet as recommended. She also faithfully did her myofunctional exercises to undo her habitual tongue thrust.

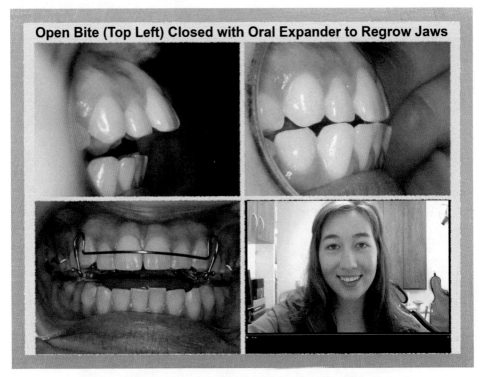

Open Bite (Top Left) Closed with Oral Expander to Regrow Jaws

Figure 20. *Severe open bite (upper left) closed with epigenetic oral appliance (lower left) which led to facial radiance (lower right).*

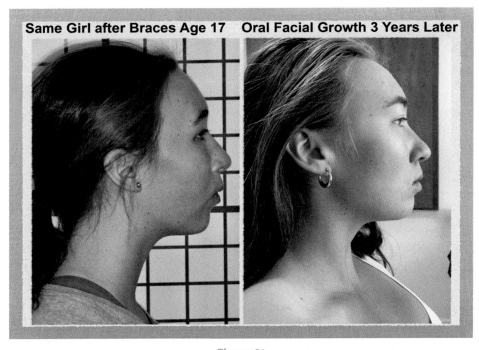

Figure 21

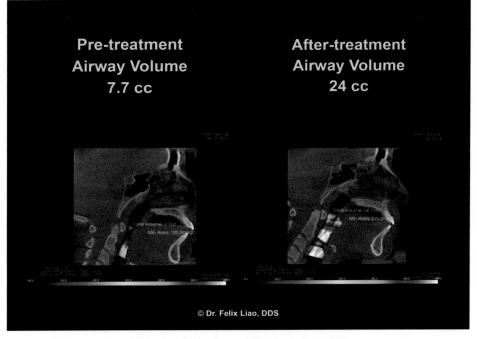

Figure 22. *HR's airway more than tripled with epigenetic oral appliance and eating healthier.*

HR's facial radiance in Figure 23 comes from the regrowth of her maxilla. Her airway tripled due to the oral appliance in combination with a healthier diet. None of this would have happened without an informed referral from chiropractors Drs. Krakos & Lim.

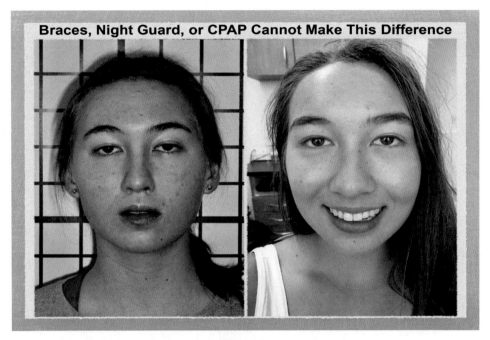

Figure 23

She has since become a part-time model and a confident young lady. She can look forward to a smooth medical-dental destiny (see Figure 17). To get this outcome, however, HR's parents did have to pay twice — once for braces and another to fix the root cause of her teeth grinding and relapse after braces: a deficient maxilla. The rest of this book will show how you too can do it right for your child from the start.

Conclusions:

- Maxilla growth is maximally important because a deficient maxilla is the start of airway obstruction and half-stunted face.
- Early recognition by parents can bring out a better face in every child with:
  - Eating a diet that promotes growth and builds bone.
  - Having guidance from a trained Airway Mouth Doctor and myofunctional therapist.
  - Seeing the red flags (next chapter) early on.

CHAPTER 2
RED FLAGS
Dental Crowding and Other Early Warnings

If better face means better health, then what does it take to achieve Best Face with top health? Most kids lose 20 baby teeth and gain 28 adult teeth by age 15. This means dental crowding is built in — unless the jaws grow sufficiently.

Teeth become bunched up when Murphy's Law takes over Nature's Plan. Let's look at crowding with a "CSI" (crime scene investigation) eye to find and arrest the culprits early on.

Crowded & Crooked Teeth: WHY?

Dental crowding is all about the jaw growth, which in turn affects the vital airway that fuels every child's sleep, learning, and growth.

Figure 24 shows a case of severely jumbled teeth, while Figure 25 shows the choked airway of the same child.

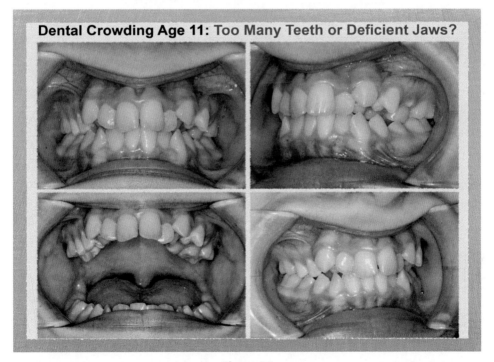

Figure 24

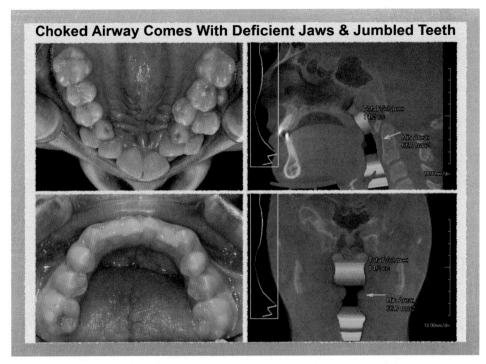

Choked Airway Comes With Deficient Jaws & Jumbled Teeth

Figure 25. *Black zones in the right CT images show the choked airway in the back of the same child's underdeveloped jaws.*

Choked airway can lead to oxygen deficiency and contribute to children's attention deficit, anxiety, depression, lower learning, and more.

What are the causes of crowding and a choked airway? The full answer is detailed in *Licensed to Thrive* (see Resources on page 94). The short answer is too little real estate — jaw growth falling short of full genetic potential.

Lower front teeth crowding, as in Figure 25, means maxilla is underdeveloped. This is a useful CSI clue. Since mandible should fit into maxilla like a foot in a shoe, the scrunched toes reflect an undersized toe box.

Growing maxilla to its full size with room for all teeth is the key to grow your child's Best Face. Like each member in a family, every tooth is entitled its seat at the table.

Dental Amputees

Dental amputees are patients with 1, 2, 4, and even 8 teeth pulled and the vacated spaces closed with braces. Pulling new teeth to make room to straighten the remaining ones is an accepted treatment for crowded teeth. "When I got to junior high school, every kid went to the orthodontist. I was just the next kid in line to get teeth pulled and braces put on," shrugged one new 62-year-old patient with chronic sinus pain and infection as well as neck and shoulder pain.

He is hardly alone. His wife also had four teeth pulled for braces. Her presenting complaints were gum recession, pain in her jaw joints, jaw clenching, and an achy left hip and tail bone that defied conventional treatment.

Dental amputation misses and aggravates Impaired Mouth Syndrome. Figure 26 shows a pair of twins. Do you prefer the face on the left or the right for your child? Remember that dental amputation is forever in that pulled teeth cannot be put back.

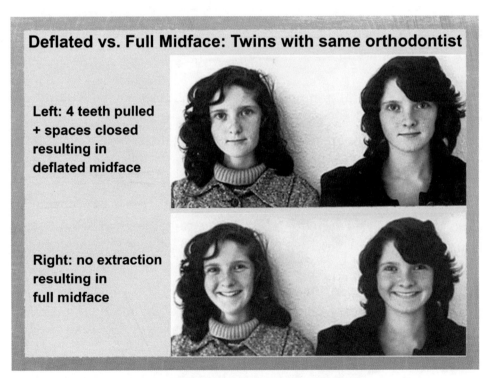

Deflated vs. Full Midface: Twins with same orthodontist

Left: 4 teeth pulled + spaces closed resulting in deflated midface

Right: no extraction resulting in full midface

Figure 26. *It took a very courageous orthodontist to publish this case study and make his point.*

In my experience as an AMD, I notice dental amputees often suffer more severe Impaired Mouth Syndrome. See chapter 4 Triple Whammy in *Relaunch Your Vitality* in References.

A Higher Bar: Best Face Before Straight Teeth

Crowding means the jaws are already too small for all the teeth and the tongue. Taking out teeth and closing the spaces makes a bad case worse, as seen in this real-life scenario from a concerned parent:

"In trying to correct a severe overbite, my parents paid for braces, and my orthodontist pulled four teeth to correct my bite. I later had my four wisdom teeth removed. Now in my 40's I have trouble breathing while sleeping and wake up exhausted. I am grinding my teeth at night and damaging my enamel and gums. I also need to see my chiropractor often.

I would like to correct the problem instead of treating the symptoms. I would also like to consult about my children, ages 12 & 9, to avoid these mistakes for them. I am convinced that braces are not a good solution, but this is all my dentist is trained in."

You can avoid dental amputation and even braces for your child by ensuring fully grown jaws. Each tooth is entitled to its plot of jaw bone in God's plan. Braces have their place for straightening teeth. Why wait until you have crowded teeth?

We need a higher standard than just straight teeth. For my granddaughter, it would be Best Face with a full set of straight teeth to bring on top health and a natural glow.

Ask your dentist if growing jaws to make Best Face is part of his or her training. Meanwhile, be on the lookout for any of the more common red flags listed in Figure 27.

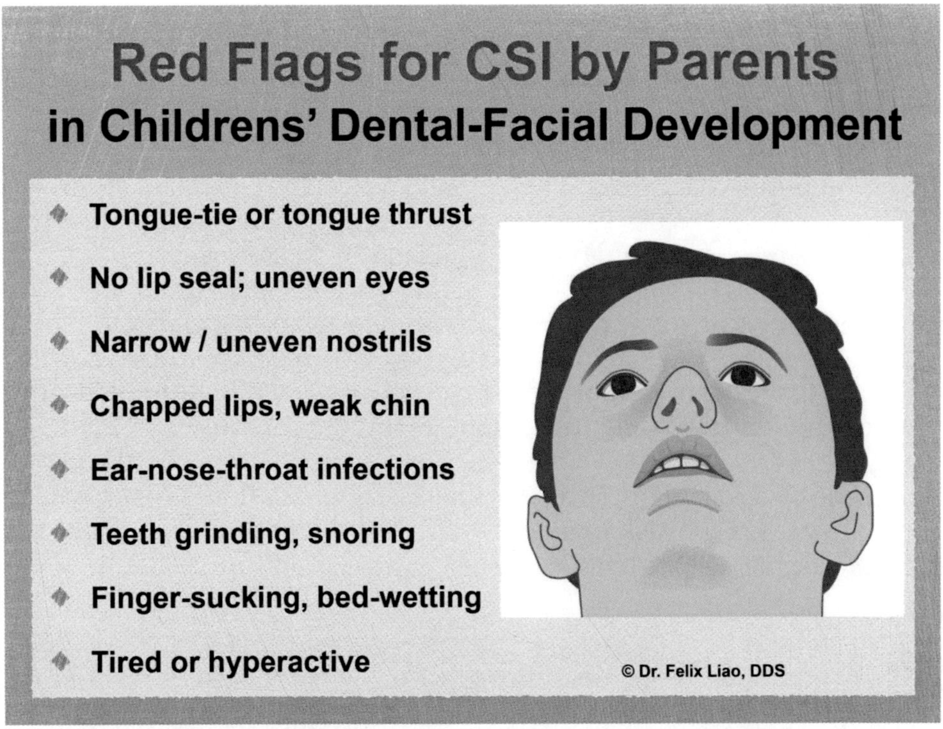

Red Flags for CSI by Parents
in Childrens' Dental-Facial Development

- **Tongue-tie or tongue thrust**
- **No lip seal; uneven eyes**
- **Narrow / uneven nostrils**
- **Chapped lips, weak chin**
- **Ear-nose-throat infections**
- **Teeth grinding, snoring**
- **Finger-sucking, bed-wetting**
- **Tired or hyperactive**

© Dr. Felix Liao, DDS

Figure 27. *Example of an Impaired Mouth in a child. This view reveals lip incompetence and asymmetry in the eyes, ears, and nostrils. CSI: Crime scene investigation.*

Frequent Red Flags

Clues that your child's dental-facial development may be taking a wrong turn (away from full genetic potential) can include but are not limited to:

- Crowded, crooked, bucked, or blocked-out teeth.
- Sad-looking face with downcast expression.
- Low energy and learning struggles.
- Waking up tired, bed wetting long past potty training.
- Prone to cavities, infections, colds and flus.
- Weak chin, slumped posture, being bullied in school.
- Little appetite, picky eater.
- Teeth grinding, thumb sucking, nail biting.
- Abnormal swallowing, such as tongue thrust, gurgling sound, grimaced face, and goose-necking.

- Chapped, peeling lips.
- Blue or purplish colored lips instead of pink.
- Hyperactive, attention deficit.
- Obesity, epilepsy, pediatric sleep apnea.

These conditions are stressful to the child as well as parents. The causes are many. Let's focus on three that are largely in your parental control: tongue-tie, epigenetics (nurturing), and healthy home cooking.

Lifelong Consequences of Tongue-Tie Undiagnosed

Behind every case of dental crowding and Impaired Mouth Syndrome lurks an undiagnosed tongue-tie, habitual mouth breathing, or both.

Tongue-tie comes in many sizes and shapes. Figure 28 shows a severe case of tongue-tie. The whitish ligament under the tongue pulls the tongue tip backward into a heart shape.

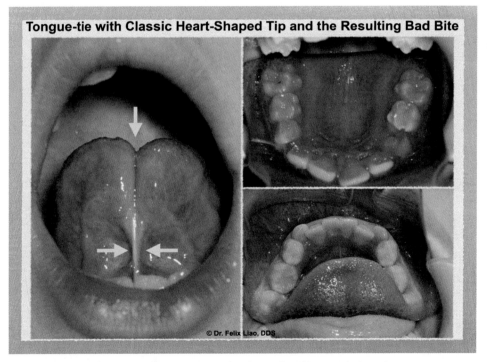

Figure 28. *Severe tongue-tie with noticeably crowded teeth.*

Tongue-tie, regardless of severity, can lead to teeth crowding because the tongue is anchored to the floor of the mouth, unable to reach the palate to stimulate maxilla growth as in breastfeeding. Failure of maxilla to reach full size leads to the same in mandible, resulting in lower front teeth crowding.

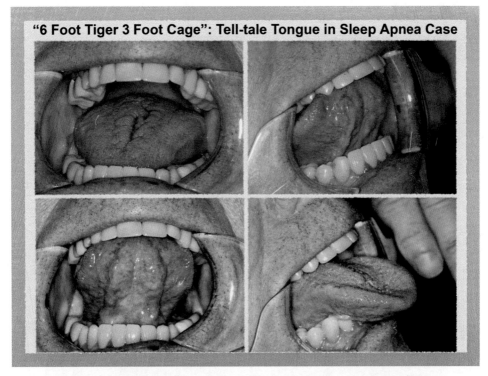

"6 Foot Tiger 3 Foot Cage": Tell-tale Tongue in Sleep Apnea Case

Figure 29. *Top left: An oversize-tongue unable to fit between the jaws (6 Foot Tiger in 3 Foot Cage). Bottom left: Tongue-tie in this case is a broad band under the tongue. Bottom right: The lack of tongue extension reflecting tongue-tie; its saucer shape comes from the pull by the broad band from underneath.*

Figure 29 shows the tongue of a man in his early 60s with medically diagnosed obstructive sleep apnea. He is a four-teeth dental amputee and sleeps with a CPAP mask. All his teeth were crowned (capped) at considerable cost, and his tongue-tie remained undiagnosed for 60 years.

When we trace this poor patient's downhill slide to the top, tongue-tie was at the starting gate. In addition to causing a bad bite, a tongue-tie can even induce the classic facial profile of a witch, as in Figure 4. A tongue-tie can be released like a longer leash, but it's never "cut out" like an appendix or extracted tooth.

Root Causes of Deficient Jaw Growth

Jaw growth at birth begins with breastfeeding and continues through the teens with eating healthy and sleeping without airway obstruction. In my view, the most pervasive causes of deficient jaw growth can include:

- Severe tongue-tie interfering with breastfeeding.
- Moderate or mild tongue-tie anchoring the tongue to the floor of the mouth instead of resting against the palate to stimulate maxilla growth.
- Improper weaning.
- Habitual mouth breathing from nasal congestion and swollen tonsils.
- Typical American diet with fast-food, take-outs, and sugar-laden drinks.

A dentist trained as an Airway Mouth Doctor (AMD) and myofunctional therapist can help parents interpret the "clues at the crime scene" and find the culprit.

The Case of PB

PB came with epileptic seizures, a long list of medications, and a deep overbite. Figures 30–36 tell his case story.

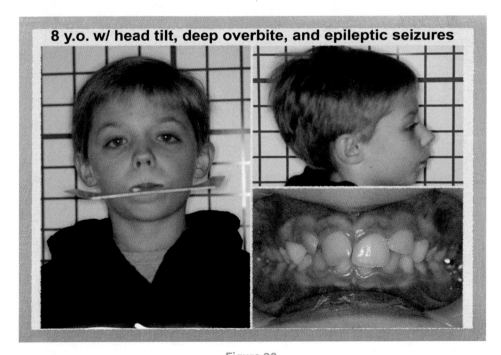

8 y.o. w/ head tilt, deep overbite, and epileptic seizures

Figure 30

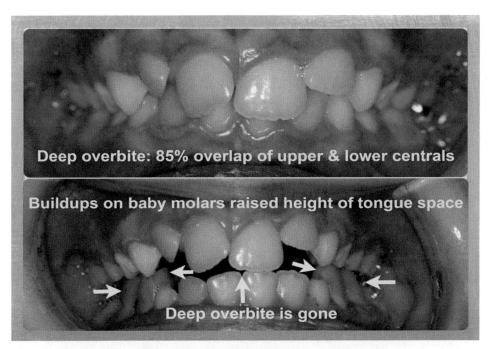

Figure 31. *Top: Deep overbite (90% overlap by upper front teeth over lowers pre-treatment. Bottom: Overbite gone after build-ups placed over lower baby molars (side arrows) with no injection or drilling needed.*

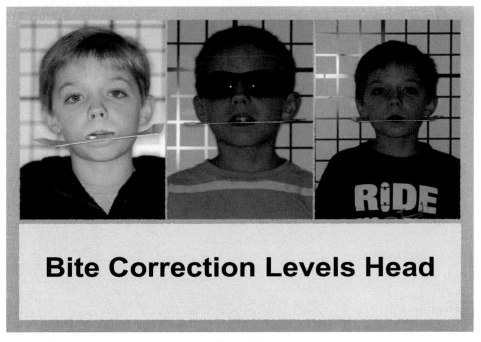

Figure 32

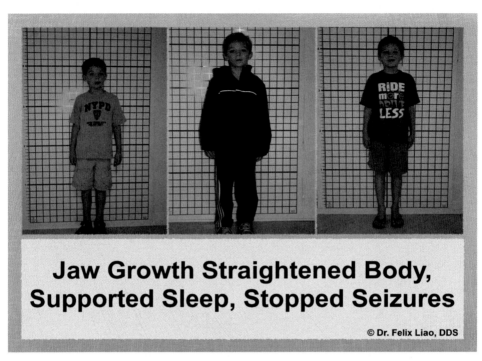

Jaw Growth Straightened Body, Supported Sleep, Stopped Seizures

© Dr. Felix Liao, DDS

Figure 33

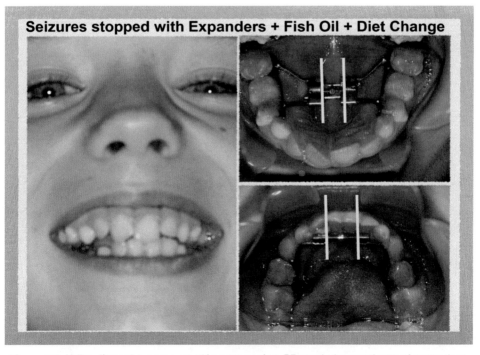

Seizures stopped with Expanders + Fish Oil + Diet Change

Figure 34. *Yellow lines show amount of jaw expansion. PB needed several sets of expanders.*

Correcting PB's overbite (one visit and without injection, as in Figure 31) and diet change (adding fish and eggs) stopped his seizures completely. Palatal expanders widened his airway, improved his sleep, straightened his head-body posture, and fueled his growth. Braces were used to line up his teeth.

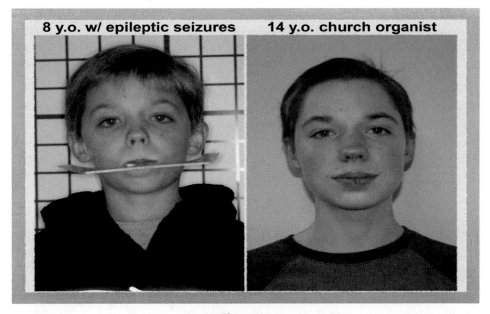

Figure 35

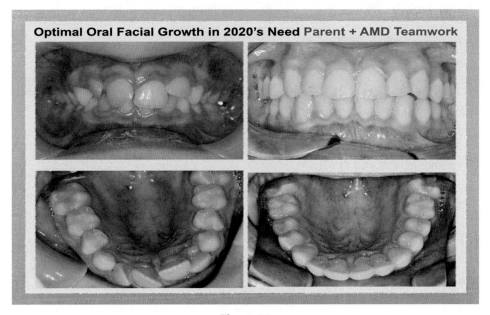

Figure 36

Looking back at PB's case, it's plausible that seizures can be connected with oxygen deprivation from airway obstruction. PB's case also offered many medical, dental, mental, and postural clues for CSI.

Airway Mouth Consultants (AMCs)

Airway Mouth Consultants (AMC) are non-dentist healthcare professionals who have training in Impaired Mouth Syndrome diagnosis and treatment. AMC can include physicians, chiropractic doctors, doctors of physical therapy, nutritionists, respiratory therapists, cranio-sacral therapists, myofunctional therapists, dental hygienists, nurses, and dental assistants, and more. AMC can provide life-changing guidance, referral, and treatment as needed.

Combining WholeHealth teamwork between AMC and AMD can make breakthroughs in many challenging cases.

Working with a trained Airway Mouth Doctor is increasingly necessary because raising kids today to full genetic potential is far more challenging than ever. That's because of ubiquitous toxic chemicals, herbicides gone wild, processed foods engineered to hook consumers, and other environmental health blockers, which we will take up in the next two chapters.

Conclusions:

- Crooked teeth, bad posture, teeth grinding, and sleep apnea all can come from the same source: deficient maxilla growth.

- Impaired Mouth Syndrome in adults arises from not seeing the red flags mentioned, and not attending to them in childhood.

- Crowded teeth is a late sign of Impaired Mouth, but it's never too late to recognize and treat.

- Extracting new teeth is a permanent and irreplaceable loss. Consider the root cause before resorting to dental amputation: an already undersized jaw and narrow airway.

- Every parent needs professional guidance and support to nurture Best Face, for which AMDs are specifically trained.

CHAPTER 3

WHOLEHEALTH TEAMWORK

The Secret Sauce to Breakthrough Outcomes

Life at birth begins with a cry to inflate the lungs and then a feeding followed by blessed sleep. This is how every one of us started in this world. Give your child what it needs and their body will thrive. Sounds sensible in a book, but it's not as simple in real life.

Thriving your child's health requires special parental attention and active work. "You can't buy good health; you have to earn it", as Dr. Joel Fuhrman MD[3] says pointedly. Your child's Best Face is *earned* by:

A. Growing his/her maxilla to full genetic potential so all 16 teeth can line up straight.

B. Partnering with a dentist trained as an Airway Mouth Doctor for guidance.

C. Seeing like-minded professionals as needed to straighten whole body health.

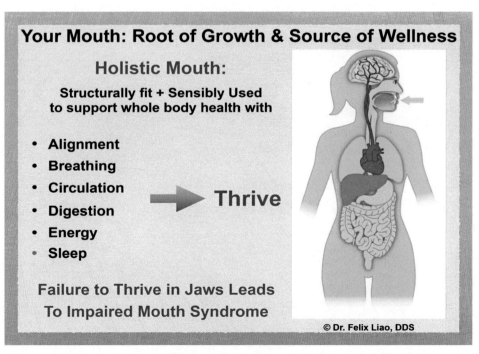

Figure 37. *Committed Parents + Trained AMDs = Best Face with Top Health.*

WholeHealth vs. Silo Mentality

WholeHealth is how the body works: all parts are interconnected, and all systems are seamlessly integrated. WholeHealth is a viewfinder zoomed out to see the Whole from head to feet, and from birth to now. Whole-Health is the opposite of tunnel vision: one specialty for each body part and missing the Whole.

With each Impaired Mouth come many clues beyond crowded teeth. PB's case in chapter 2 came with co-symptoms besides crowded teeth: epilepsy, head tilt, stunted growth, tired-looking face, and challenged learning.

WholeHealth means seeing past the typical medical, dental, and mental silos of *just* dental crowding, just neck pain, just seizure, and just snoring, and so on. WholeHealth in clinical practice means knowing how to put all parts and systems back to a working Whole.

Heading off Impaired Mouth & Chronic Pain Proactively

Mouth structure and jaw alignment are foundational to whole body health. Dr. Mariano Rocabado, PhD in Physical Therapy, states that "100% of headaches and neck pain has malocclusion (bad bite). And that is bi-directional."

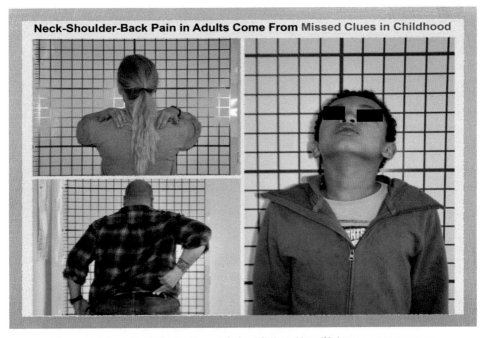

Figure 38. *Impaired Mouth diagnosis in childhood has lifelong consequences.*

I agree completely. If you have a bad bite, you'll have neck pain, and when you have recurring neck pain despite treatment, look for a bad bite.

A case of such collaboration between a postural-restoration physical therapist (PRPT) Heather Carr, DPT, and an AMD is seen in Figures 39 and 40.

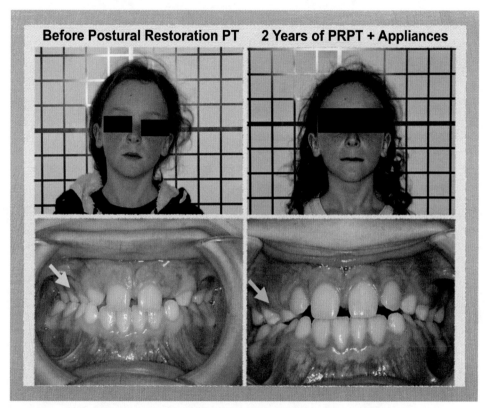

Figure 39. *Left: Pre-treatment head tilt and cross bite (yellow arrow). Right: Head tilt and cross bite gone (green arrow).*

The boy's head tilt came from his cross bite rooted in an undersized maxilla. Combining postural restoration physical therapy and a maxilla growth appliance made the differences seen in Figures 39 and 40.

Compare eye levels and head lift before and after treatment in Figure 40. This is how WholeHealth works in childhood to head off neck and back pain later. These positive outcomes have a prerequisite: the patient's doctor/therapist must know about Impaired Mouth Syndrome and Holistic Mouth Solutions.

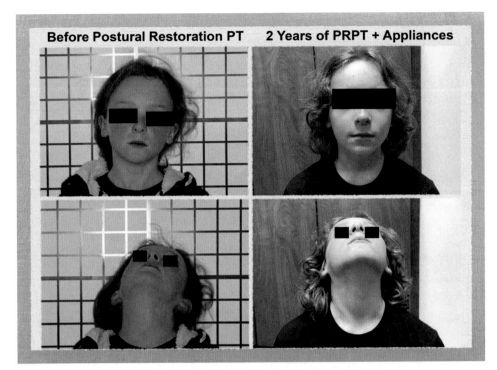

Figure 40. *Postural Restoration Physical Therapy (PRPT) plus oral appliance normalized his head posture.*

Epigenetic Blockers of Jaw Development

A couch potato can change their body shape by taking up running, swimming, dancing, and eating healthier. Same person, same genes, yet new physical body.

"Epigenetics is the study of how your behaviors and environment can cause changes that affect the way your genes work", explains the CDC[4].

Think of epigenetics as "nurture" — parental attention to red flags during jaw growth and facial development. Epigenetic factors like lip seal and a bone-building diet can tip a child's growth toward Best Face within her or his genes, instead of the one in Figures 11 and 12.

Conversely, crowded teeth, weak chin, or flat mid-face arise from epigenetic blockers stopping full genetic potential, such as:

A. **Environmental pollutants:** greenhouse gases, acid rain, plastics, pharmaceutical residues in tap water, etc.

B. **Processed/packaged foods** loaded with added sugars, salts, fats and laced with preservatives, herbicide residues, and other chemicals.

C. **Tongue-tie** leading to abnormal swallows 2,000 times a day for years.

D. **Habitual mouth breathing** from chronic nasal congestion and gut inflammation.

A structurally Impaired Mouth has these as major causes. Getting educated is the first step. The next is seeing a trained AMD for Impaired Mouth diagnosis and WholeHealth solution.

An epigenetic oral appliance in combination with bodywork and a bone-building diet can make up where nature and nurture fall short. Figure 41 shows such a case.

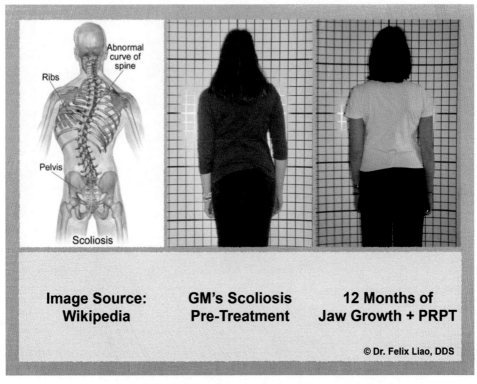

Image Source: Wikipedia	GM's Scoliosis Pre-Treatment	12 Months of Jaw Growth + PRPT

© Dr. Felix Liao, DDS

Figure 41. *Scoliosis is the abnormal curvature of the spine in children and a cause of pain in adults. Compare uneven shoulders, hips, and the space between her right arm and body in the center and right images.*

Scoliosis Breakthrough with WholeHealth Teamwork

GM, age 14, was referred to me for scoliosis by a postural-restoration Doctor of Physical Therapy (DPT) who had heard me speak on Impaired Mouth Syndrome. This is a shining example of WholeHealth teamwork.

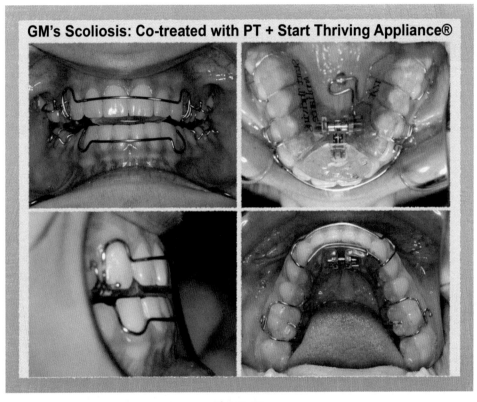

Figure 42

Scoliosis would have been none of my business when I was still a tooth-centered dentist. Since becoming an AMD with WholeHealth awareness, I now do my part to diagnose and treat Impaired Mouth in concert with like-minded body alignment professionals.

WholeHealth is our common aim. That means every doctor and therapist need to know how the mouth is connected to the spine, the organs, and the Whole, and vice versa.

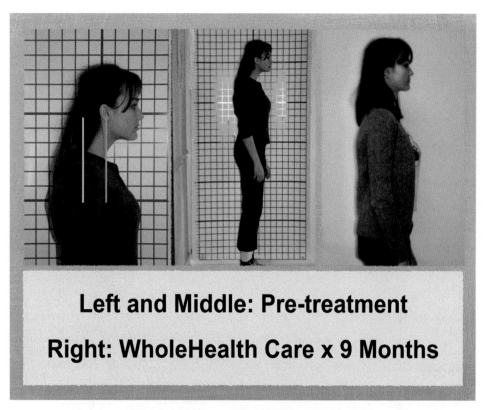

Left and Middle: Pre-treatment

Right: WholeHealth Care x 9 Months

Figure 43. *A breakthrough outcome from WholeHealth collaboration.*

GM's full compliance drives her progress as follows: doing all her therapy exercises, wearing her oral appliance 14–16 hours a day, and eating a bone-building diet. You can see GM recounting her progress through the link *Follow Case Progress* in Resources on page 94.

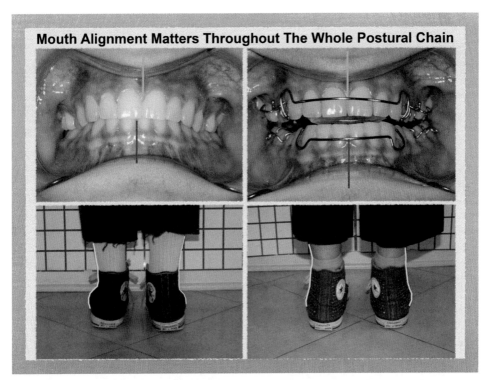

Figure 44. *Left: Dental midlines off and flat feet with inward arch collapse (pronation). Right: Impaired Mouth treatment plus PRPT improved feet pronation in 12 months.*

The greater part of the credit goes to Noelle Ekonomou, DPT, who recognized the mouth's contribution to scoliosis and fine-tuned GM's treatment while this AMD plays second violin. Figures 43–45 show the results of teamwork between an AMD and DPT.

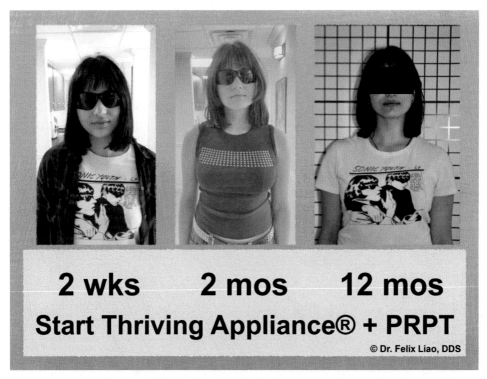

2 wks   2 mos   12 mos

Start Thriving Appliance® + PRPT

© Dr. Felix Liao, DDS

Figure 45. *The horizontal line on the same T-shirt becomes more level from left to right.*

Combining multiple areas of expertise with the same WholeHealth mission can create breakthrough outcomes in cases not previously helped by "best in my silo" treatment. Putting the patient back to a functional Whole is the whole point of WholeHealth teamwork.

Braces vs. Appliance the WholeHealth Way

Braces move teeth like boxcars on railroads, while expander appliances work on the rail bed, i.e., jaw length, width, and height to make Best Face. While braces can straighten teeth, Best Face grows maxilla fully to make room for all teeth, and for airway to widen in both the nose and the throat.

Another part of the secret sauce to success is how an epigenetic oral appliance is engineered to target deficiencies. Start Thriving Appliance® is designed with 3D Jaw Diagnostics® to precisely target what's off and where. With this appliance, parents also receive WholeHealth guidance (re: stuffy nose, head tilt, tongue-tie) and a bone-building diet to help fully grow the maxilla. In this way, success is baked into each Start Thriving Appliance individually.

"Seasonal Affective Disorder Improved"

SA, age 16, came with popping jaw joints "for as long as [she] can remember," plus jaw clenching in her sleep. Her health history included braces three years earlier, and medications for ADHD and depression for six years.

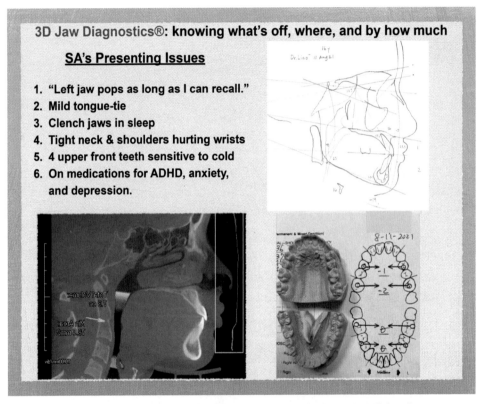

Figure 46. *3D Jaw Diagnostics® reveals SA's Impaired Mouth deficiencies: undersized maxilla (lower right image) leads to cramped space for her tongue and choked airway (black zone lower left image).*

Straight white teeth with choked airway falls short of WholeHealth success. Looking good alone is not good enough for natural health and wellness in adults and children alike. Before her Start Thriving Appliance treatment, SA's maxilla and airway were both too narrow and her "three-foot cage" too squashed in length and width to support adequate oxygen supply to her brain, as shown in Figure 46.

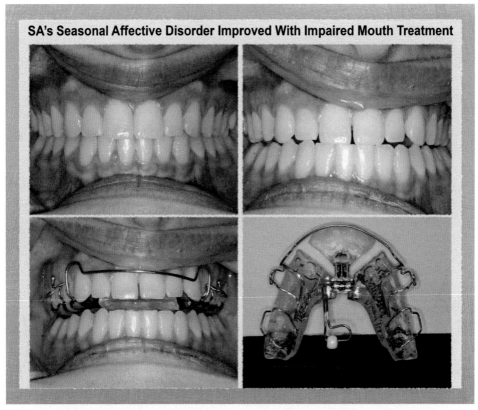

Figure 47. *Top left: Pre-treatment; lower left and right: Start Thriving Appliance® in and out of mouth; Upper right: Lower jaw freed from entrapment in mid-treatment because of maxilla regrowth. Treatment is ongoing.*

SA reported sleeping better after three weeks of treatment with a maxilla appliance in the fall. The gaps between the three parts of her appliance shown in Figure 47 (lower right image) reflects her maxilla growth in four months. Her comments throughout the winter included:

- "Breathing has gotten easier."
- "Dreaming getting more vivid."
- "Seasonable Affective Disorder (SAD) improved," which her dad confirmed: "noticeable difference with mood in February."

Targeting SA's maxilla helped to improve her mental health through deeper sleep. As a result, SA's anti-depressant medication has been cut in half from 20 to 10 mg in seven months. "We are very excited about the drop", emailed her mom.

GM's and SA's cases illustrate the essence of WholeHealth — the mouth is connected to the Whole, mind and body, through airway and alignment. Yet, this obvious fact is hugely missing in today's healthcare system. This calls for cross-training among AMDs and all healthcare professionals to better treat tilted head, scoliosis, pronated feet, and mood disorders. See Cross-Training Summit. See item #6 in Resources on page 94.

Conclusions:

- Proper alignment of the head, jaws, and bite over the neck is foundational for the whole body to work better.

- Airway is not optional, neither is Alignment. That's why AMDs and all healthcare professionals need to work as a WholeHealth team.

- Cross-training in WholeHealth is a necessary foundation for Whole-Health teamwork.

- The secret sauce to treatment success has 3 parts: educated parents, WholeHealth teamwork, and a trained AMD.

- See a trained Airway Mouth Doctor for evaluation by age nine and align your child's whole-body posture by age 12–15 if possible.

CHAPTER 4
"WHAT'S FOR DINNER?"
Fresh Home Cooking to Grow Your Child's Best Face

How's a busy working mom or dad supposed to figure out seven dinners a week, 52 weeks a year for decades?! Yet what you put on the table can either thrive your child's jaw growth or short-change it.

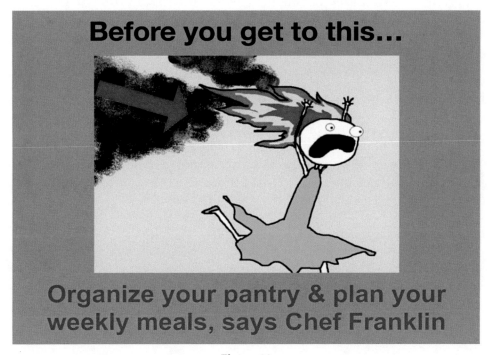

Before you get to this...

Organize your pantry & plan your weekly meals, says Chef Franklin

Figure 48

Fresh home cooking is foundational to Best Face, in my opinion. This is worth repeating: Best Face is *earned* with parental nurture and professional attention, not ordered online with a credit card. Meal and grocery deliveries do not come with Grandma's TLC, or yours.

Best Face with both jaws reaching full genetic potential is a tall order. It's 15 years of vigilant parenting on food sourcing and freshness to empower optimal facial growth. Best Face is quite a commitment!

Best Face takes more than filling the belly with just any food. What your child eats shapes the jaws and her or his face. Your nurturing is the most powerful epigenetic factor of them all.

Nurturing means your personal caring and presence, but the outcome is oh-so-worth it. This chapter covers fresh home cooking to limit the environmental toxins and added sugars and hormones increasingly present in our foods.

3 Parenting Musts to Grow Best Face

Growing your child's Best Face begins with breastfeeding whenever humanly possible, the absence of a tongue-tie, nasal breathing, and sound nutrition. It continues with these three essential parenting practices:

1. Provide tasty and healthy meals made fresh at home.
2. Model healthy eating and lifestyle habits.
3. Seek guidance and support from a trained AMD.

Let's look into why.

Toxic Chemicals, Head Size, & Jaw Growth

The mouth is the admission office between our outside and inside. The absence of modern toxins is crucial to healthy growth and full facial development. Here's the bad news you must know:

- Fetal head circumference[5] is smaller in the offspring of women with higher levels of PCBs[6] and organo-chlorine pesticides[7] (industrial products or chemicals).

- 287 industrial chemicals and pollutants (180 of them are cancer-causing in humans or animals) were found in the umbilical cord blood of newborns in the US, as reported in this 2004 EWG study[8].

- "Documented links between prenatal exposure to environmental chemicals span the life course and include impacts on fertility and pregnancy, neurodevelopment, and cancer", warns International Federation of Gynecology & Obstetrics in its 2015 report[9].

- "Weed Killer Found in All Kids' Cereals Sampled", reported EWG in 2018[10]. "... almost all of the samples tested by EWG had residues of glyphosate at levels higher than what EWG scientists consider protective of children's health with an adequate margin of safety."

- Pharmaceuticals pass through water treatment, says US Geological Survey[11].

Figure 49 shows why you may not want to take tap water and clean air for granted.

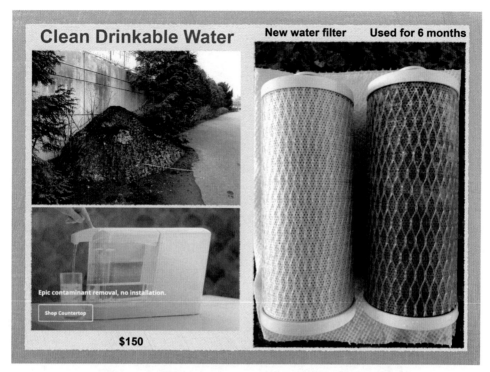

Figure 49. **Top left:** *Soot-covered snow after one week in metro Washington DC.* **Right:** *A new water filter vs. one used for 6 months.*

Healthy children are products of healthy parents AND Mother Earth. See *Licensed To Thrive*, chapters 5–13 for more details.

Our Ancestors' Collective Wisdom

Regardless of ethnic origin, our ancestors learned to live in harmony with Planet Earth. They ate naturally grown foods and developed regional diets that sustained their offspring until recently. We are indebted to Sally Fallon for starting Weston A. Price Foundation to guide parents, and their doctors and dentists, in the 21st century. See Figures 16 & 17 and Resources on page 95.

Parents can adopt this collective wisdom to help their kids achieve Best Face, then use epigenetic expanders to stimulate further jaw growth as needed.

The faces of typical indigenous Taiwanese people and their diets are shown in Figures 50 and 51. A typical lunch includes fish caught fresh off the beach that morning, wrapped in banana leaf, and baked in a charcoal oven dug into the ground. Such epigenetics show up on their faces and dental arches.

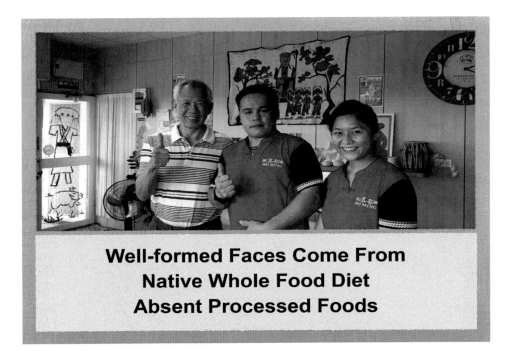

**Well-formed Faces Come From
Native Whole Food Diet
Absent Processed Foods**

Figure 50. Taiwan natives (center and right) grew up without dental floss, pediatrician, and orthodontists. They have better-formed faces than this author (left) who grew up eating semi-Americanized "city diet".

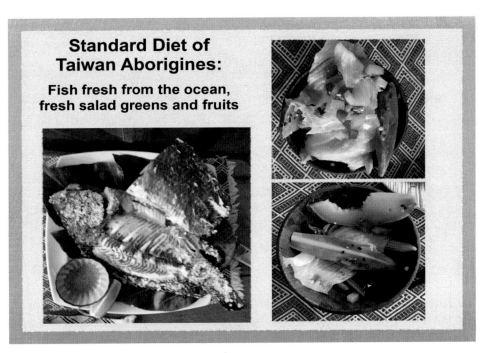

**Standard Diet of
Taiwan Aborigines:**

**Fish fresh from the ocean,
fresh salad greens and fruits**

Figure 51

Whole Food Diet

Cooking carefully sourced fresh whole foods at home is the best way to limit environmental toxins into your child's body. It gives you control over water quality, preservatives, fixatives, herbicides, emulsifiers, and salt, fat, and sugar overload. This is not possible with fast, processed, and commercially prepared and delivered foods.

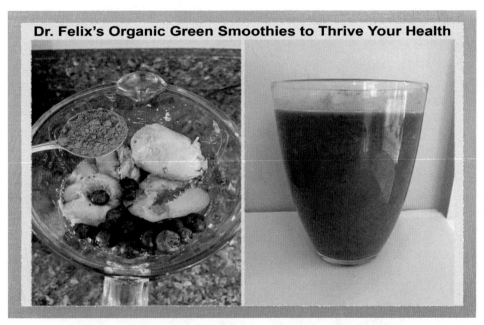

Dr. Felix's Organic Green Smoothies to Thrive Your Health

Figure 52. *Ingredients: Fresh peach, blueberries, avocado, organic chocolate powder, and over a bed of arugula in a blender with filtered water. Mix and match what's in season, local, and fresh.*

Long shelf life and fresh whole foods are mutually exclusive. When you cook at home, you can ensure you are including bone-building ingredients to help grow your child's maxilla, mandible, and face.

If you find cooking to be a chore, or if you just don't know what to cook, check out Chef Franklin's *Cook2Thrive* website (based on my book *Licensed to Thrive*) to help with organizing your pantry and meal planning. Here's a post by Chef Franklin, my son:

"What's for dinner?" I asked my girlfriend one afternoon.

"Cereal," she said. "What?!" I kept it to myself: cereal for dinner?

"Why don't WE cook something?" I made a simple offer instead.

"Cereal is faster," she said dismissively.

I then told her what we'd be making. She abruptly changed her mind: "How can I help you?"

Together, we made turkey meat balls, smashed cucumbers with ginger, scallions, and steamed rice. It was yummy, and our kids loved it!

Yes, it does take some preparation and a desire for better. But you can't get conversation, laughter, creativity, and family fun out of a box.

The next time "what's for dinner?" comes up, consider enlisting a family member, or call up a friend, to share in the joy of cooking and sharing a meal and washing dishes together.

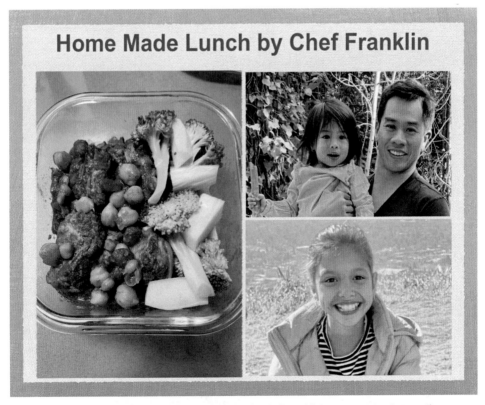

Home Made Lunch by Chef Franklin

Figure 53. Left: *Ingredients include braised ribs, chick peas, steam broccoli, and parental TLC. You too can make healthy foods tasty at home for your kids.* **Right:** *Chef Franklin with Camila and step daughter SDH.*

Consider replacing your take-outs and delivered meals with thoughtfully chosen foods made fresh at home. Start with baby steps going from one day a week to two and three and so on. Chef Franklin's food budget for his family of four was $450–600 per month in 2021 before inflation. "It's not worth it for me to resort to junk food", said Chef Franklin. "Lots of work but lots of reward." See Figures 68 & 69 in chapter 6.

The kids can tell. Here's what happened at lunch as reported by 11 year-old SDH, Chef Franklin's step daughter:

> New classmate at lunch on day 1 in new school year: *"Are you on a special diet?"*
> SDH: *No, why?*
> One classmate: *Your lunch just looks "healthy".*
> Another classmate: *Want to try a fruit roll-up?*
> SDH: *Okay, I've never tried one before.*
> Classmate: *What? Really?*
> SDH: *I don't like it.*
> Classmate: *What's wrong with you?*
> SDH: *I just don't like eating things that taste like plastic.*

Your child's Best Face depends critically on what you feed them. Fresh home cooking professionally designed is now available to help you and your child thrive. See Resources on page 94. Then team up with an AMD.

Conclusions:

- Cooking fresh food at home is a vital parenting skill and Best Face necessity. This is where you as a parent "earn" top health and Best Face for your child.

- Parental awareness plus professional guidance by a trained AMD can bring out your kid's Best Face with natural glow.

CHAPTER 5

BRINGING ON BEST FACE
How Success Is Baked In

The mouth is to humans what roots are to plants, as I wrote in *Licensed to Thrive.* In Dr. Paul Chek's *Totem Pole Hierarchy of Survival Reflexes* (2015), breathing and eating are on the very top, as Figure 54 shows. Whether to survive or to thrive, the mouth has the starting role. That's why every parent wanting Best Face needs an Airway Mouth Doctor (AMD).

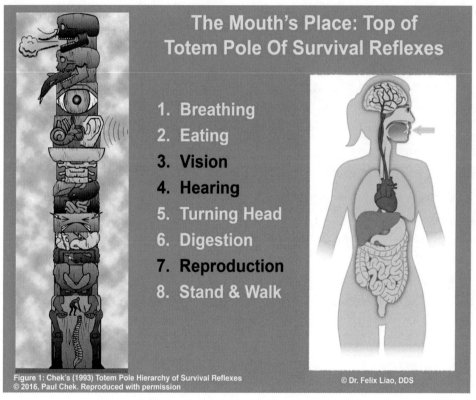

Figure 1: Chek's (1993) Totem Pole Hierarchy of Survival Reflexes
© 2016, Paul Chek. Reproduced with permission

© Dr. Felix Liao, DDS

Figure 54. *Oral contributions include items 1, 2, 5, 6, and 8.*

A trained AMD is a Guide (think Gandalf and Yoda) to parents in quest of their children's Best Face. Such guidance can include, but is not limited to, the preparation of the maternal environment, weaning properly, and preventing and detecting flat midface, weak chin, and Impaired Mouth.

Preparation of Maternal Environment

An AMD can help women of child-bearing age with Holistic Mouth care while leaving medical care to their attending physicians as follows:

- **Pre-conception:** Prepare an optimal incubator inside the mom-to-be a year in advance if possible. Evaluation and treatment for an Impaired Mouth can remove oral contributions to back pain, insomnia, hormonal dysregulation, and more.

- **Pregnancy:** Widening the airway and aligning head-jaws-spine can reduce birth trauma to both the newborn and the mom. Ensure mom's proper alignment, breathing, circulation, nutrition, and sleep by seeing her healthcare professional plus an AMD.

- **Post-delivery:** Breastfeeding provides more than optimal nutrition for the newborn. Check with a qualified infant-feeding specialist or myofunctional therapist if tongue-tie is an issue with latching.

Breastfeeding stimulates maxilla growth. Bottle feeding, while necessary at times, comes without this benefit unless the bottle nipple can mimic the real one.

Difficulty with breastfeeding from birth to age four can be helped by a sensorimotor feeding assessment. "It is best if these professionals also have TOTs (tethered oral tissues) and myofunctional therapy training", says Hallie Bulkin, Certified Orofacial Myologist and Feeding Specialist.

If no difficulty, then an assessment by an AMD or a myofunctional therapist at age four is a good proactive step to head off forces shaping Impaired Mouth.

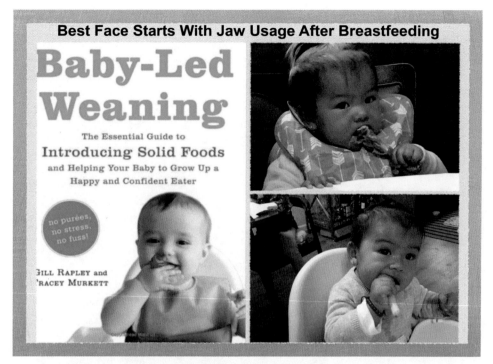

Figure 55. *Crunching on whole foods helps stimulate jaw growth with muscle action, compared to typical mush called "baby food" in a jar loaded with sugar and other additives.*

Weaning Properly

Done right, weaning leads to normal gut health and immune system maturation. Done wrong, it can result in multiple ear and respiratory infections. Repeated antibiotics can impair a good gut microbiome. Worse yet, serious gut disorders and lifelong allergies to certain foods can follow. *Baby-Led Weaning* shown in Figure 56 is another essential parenting practice toward Best Face.

Avoid Pacifiers

Avoiding the use of a pacifier is crucial if you want to avoid crowded teeth, narrow jaws, and a choked airway. Try this yourself: Pucker your lips and suck in your cheeks. This sucking pressure from a pacifier will induce a narrower maxilla over time.

A narrower maxilla leads to Impaired Mouth Syndrome. If you have already started pacifiers, consider immediate stop and consult an ΛMD or myofunctional therapist.

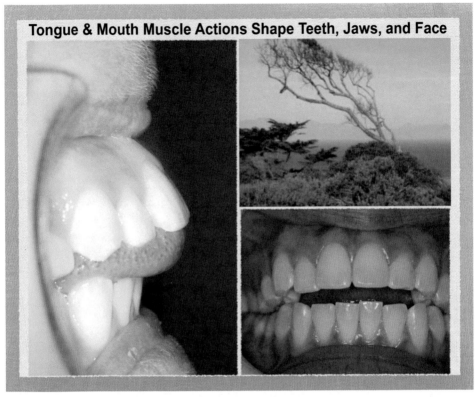

Figure 56. *Myofunctional therapy can proactively help avoid this relapse after braces.*

Mouth muscles are powerful shapers of the face through normal daily functions such as swallowing, chewing, drinking, speaking, smiling, singing, and more. As Figure 57 shows, myofunctional therapy can help normalize these muscle actions to promote optimal dental-facial development.

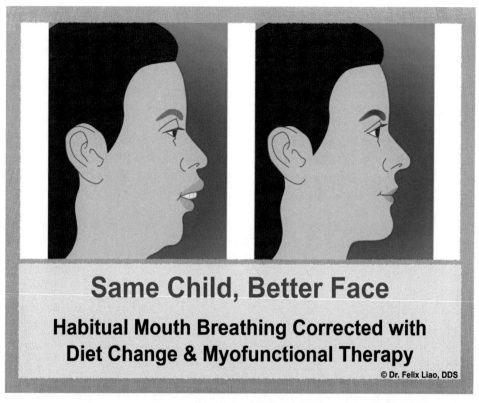

Same Child, Better Face

Habitual Mouth Breathing Corrected with Diet Change & Myofunctional Therapy

© Dr. Felix Liao, DDS

Figure 57

More Red Flags: Facial Asymmetry

As your child gets into kindergarten age, watch for head tilt and facial asymmetry — signs that the face is not level and square as shown in Figure 27 in chapter 2:

- One eye or mouth corner higher
- Uneven nostrils
- One side of face narrower
- One ear more flared
- Tilted head
- One shoulder lower
- One arm or foot more forward

Left unattended, these red flags can lead to chronic pain and fatigue in adult years. Your AMD can be your Guide and Gatekeeper to your child's Best Face. Myofunctional therapists, Airway Mouth Consultants, physical therapists, cranio-sacral therapists, chiropractic doctors and physicians all can be helpful if they are cross-trained in WholeHealth integration of mind, body, and mouth, as cases in this book have shown.

Mother's Guilt

With all this new awareness, some of you may feel a mother's guilt about wrong choices made in the past. That can include advice taken from doctor(s) who didn't practice WholeHealth.

Understand that doctors can be victims too. Some holes in their training are just coming to light. As my mentor Dr. Braden Stack was fond of saying, "Progress in healthcare is made one dead chairman at a time."

Here's how one mom worked to bring on her daughter's Best Face despite all the chairmen still alive.

The Case of LH

LH came to me at age nine because her mom, Katie, was familiar with the "clues at the crime scene," since she herself was already in treatment for impaired mouth.

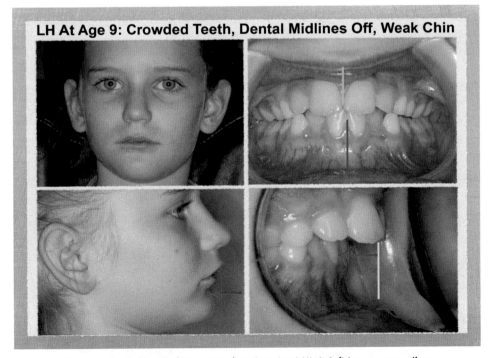

LH At Age 9: Crowded Teeth, Dental Midlines Off, Weak Chin

Figure 58. *Weak chin (red arrows) deviated to LH's left (blue vs. green line upper right) and crowded teeth are both caused by her deficient maxilla.*

3D Jaw Diagnostics®

A space by definition has three dimensions: side-to-side, front-to-back, and mouth floor to palatal roof. So does the tongue's "home office" space between the two jaws.

3D Jaw Diagnostics® can reveal which of the three dimension(s) is/are deficient or excessive, and by how much, as Figure 59 shows. That's how each Start Thriving Appliance® is custom designed to target deficiencies.

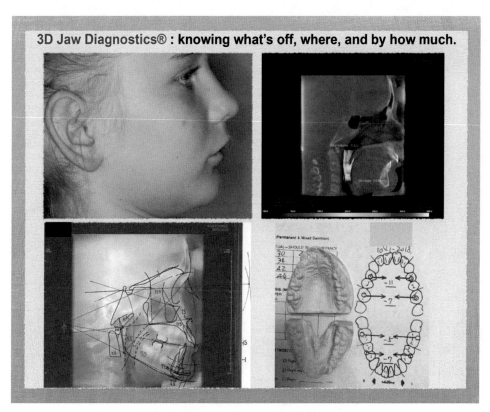

Figure 59. *3D Jaw Diagnostics® drives every Start Thriving Appliance design, including LH's.*

Figure 60 shows the resulting difference on the same day.

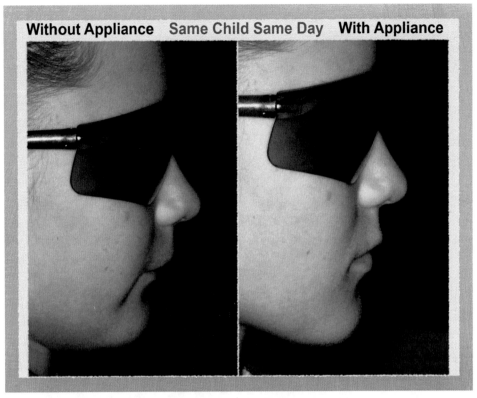

Without Appliance   Same Child Same Day   With Appliance

Figure 60. *3D Jaw Diagnostics® drives every*
Start Thriving Appliance design, including LH's.

LH benefited from an informed and committed mom who was both a craniosacral therapist and a Weston A. Price Foundation member following the Nourishing Traditions Diet (see Resources on page 95). Combining that WholeHealth base with a well-designed epigenetic oral appliance can do wonders, as Figures 61 and 62 show.

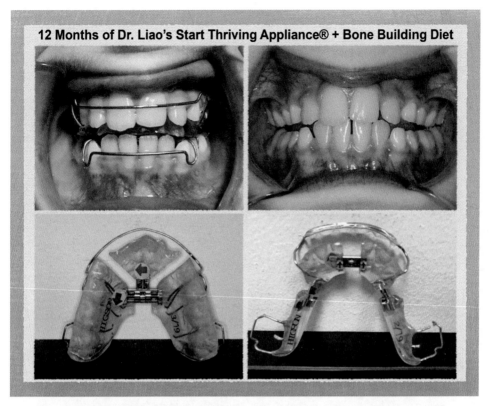

12 Months of Dr. Liao's Start Thriving Appliance® + Bone Building Diet

Figure 61. *Upper left: Appliances in place; Upper right: Lower crowding gone, while maxilla still needs further growth. Lower left and right: Gaps between appliance segments show amount and directions of jaw growth provided by LH's appliances.*

The Key to Outstanding Outcomes

Success is baked into LH's Best Face because:

1. Mom saw the red flags of weak chin and crowded lower front teeth.

2. Mom provided fresh home cooking based on Nourishing Traditions Diet (see Resources on page 95).

3. Mom teamed up with an AMD for guidance and targeted treatment.

4. Mom drove 3.5 hours each way every six weeks for four years to bring her daughters LH and RH for follow-ups.

Figures 62 and 63 as well as Figures 13 and 14 show the Best Faces "earned" by Mama Katie who is 100% supported by Papa Ted.

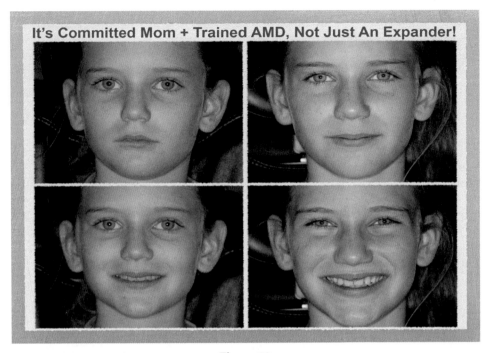

Figure 62

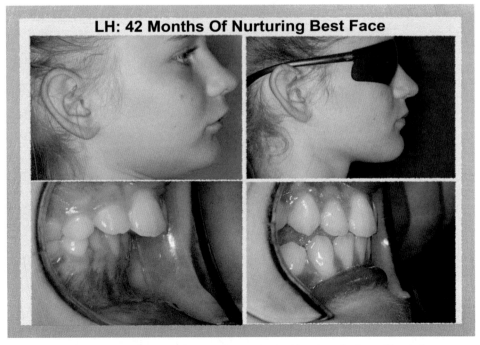

Figure 63. *LH's treatment is on-going as she had just lost the last of her baby teeth and all her adult teeth are still coming up at the time of this photo.*

As to LH's weak chin, Figure 63 shows what a committed parent teaming up with an AMD can do. You can see further progress of LH and Mama Katie by clicking *Follow Case Progress* link in Resources on page 94.

Conclusions:

- A full set of healthy teeth in a fully developed set of jaws is the key to your child's Best Face.

- The earlier, the better, but it's never too late to recognize and attend to the red flags.

- Educated and committed parents teaming up with a trained AMD can do wonders together to bring on Best Face.

CHAPTER 6
FROM DUCKLING TO SWAN
Partner with Your AMD to Make Magic

In summary, your child's Best Face is founded on a fully developed maxilla with room for all 16 teeth in combination with nasal breathing full-time. Crowded teeth show up when jaw growth falls short. The next case shows again how an educated parent and a trained AMD can make magic together.

Duckling to Swan

Dr. SN, a trained naturopath, home-school teacher, and dentist, had just started her AMD Training when she noticed her daughter SZ, age 11, was waking up tired, easily distracted, unable to focus on schoolwork, moody, and her singing was affected — which all came soon after starting braces.

Doctor Mom connected the dots and recognized Impaired Mouth Syndrome. She then stopped braces and started Start Thriving Appliances to grow SZ's jaws instead of straightening teeth. Figures 64 and 65 show the progress 10 months later without the use of braces.

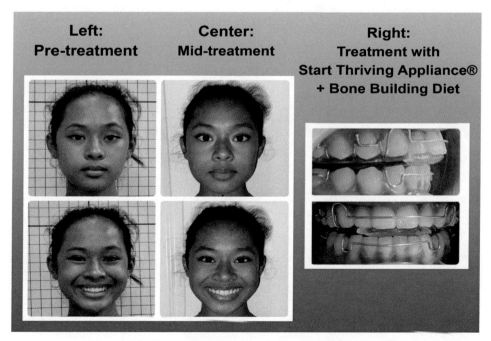

Figure 64. *Photos and permission to share courtesy of Dr. SN.*

**The Case of SZ: 10 Months Of
Start Thriving Appliance® + Bone Building Diet**

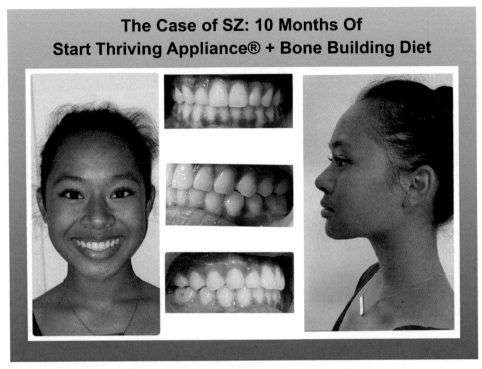

Figure 65. *No braces have been used since starting appliance treatment.*

This is not a blanket indictment of braces. Responding appropriately to symptoms after starting braces by an observant mom knowing her options is the point.

Starting targeted treatment based on WholeHealth and 3D Jaw Diagnostics before a child's growth spurt can turn an average duckling into a stand-out swan. That's the takeaway.

In addition to winning regional speech and debate competitions to qualify for the national, SZ enjoyed such comments from friends and relatives:

- "I swear once you got your braces off, not only has your face really changed but also your posture."

- "What happened to you in the last year because you don't look the same?"

- "Your smile is literal perfection"

- "Did you get a nose job?"

- "Are your teeth fake?"

Bringing on Best Face is parenting joy. Managing Impaired Mouth symptoms is not.

WholeHealth Magic

WholeHealth means empowering and restoring all bodily systems into working order, starting with the airway and the maxilla. The magic is in the logic of WholeHealth physiology (how the body works), not just an oral appliance. Again, cross-training in WholeHealth and Impaired Mouth Syndrome can be pivotal.

In a fully grown maxilla, teeth will align naturally with the normal use of lips, cheeks, and tongue. "Normal" here means no stuffy nose from congestive diet, and no tongue-tie, no tongue thrust, and no abnormal swallows. SZ checked all the boxes as a debater and singer. Her Start Thriving Appliance gave her maxilla the targeted stimulus needed to grow to its full potential.

The benefits in SZ's case include better sleep, waking up rested, greater ease with schoolwork and life, spontaneous joy, and singing with clear precision again. Use the *Follow Case Progress* link in Resources on page 94 to hear SZ telling her story and watching her sing high notes.

Best Face Needs Full-Sized Jaws

Regrowing deficient jaws starts with sound nutrition and an oral appliance in Phase I. Use braces in Phase II to straighten those teeth that still need it. Appliance work makes braces easier and faster and, in some cases, not needed.

Why Jaws Fail to Thrive Enough for All Teeth to Fit In Naturally

- ◆ **Birth Trauma: Cranial Strain**

- ◆ **Tongue-tie & Hypothyroid**

- ◆ **Air & Water Contaminants**

- ◆ **Typical American Diet Rich in**

  - ◆ **Herbicides, Pesticides**

  - ◆ **Hormones, Antibiotics**

- ◆ **Habitual Mouth Breathing**

- ◆ **No AMD Trained To See & Treat**

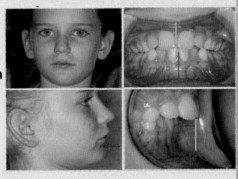

Figure 66. *For more information, see* **Licensed to Thrive**, *chapters 5–10.*

"Pediatric obstructive sleep apnea in non-obese children is a disorder of oral facial growth."

Huang & Guilleminault, Pediatric Obstructive Sleep Apnea and the Critical Role of Oral Facial Growth: Evidences. *Frontiers in Neurology* 3 (2012) PMID: 23346072

An Airway Mouth Doctor (AMD) can help you take charge of oral facial growth

© Dr. Felix Liao, DDS

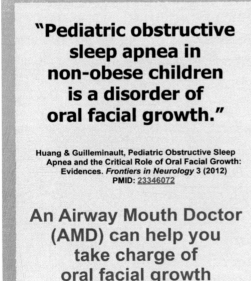

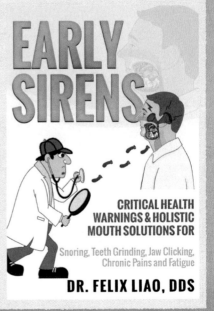

EARLY SIRENS

CRITICAL HEALTH WARNINGS & HOLISTIC MOUTH SOLUTIONS FOR

Snoring, Teeth Grinding, Jaw Clicking, Chronic Pains and Fatigue

DR. FELIX LIAO, DDS

Figure 67

A Simple Roadmap

"Rarely does treating the symptoms result in a healthy child," as Dr. Ben Mirgaglia stated so eloquently in this book's Foreword. Ensuring sound sleep with wide airway and balanced nutrition is the key to Best Face.

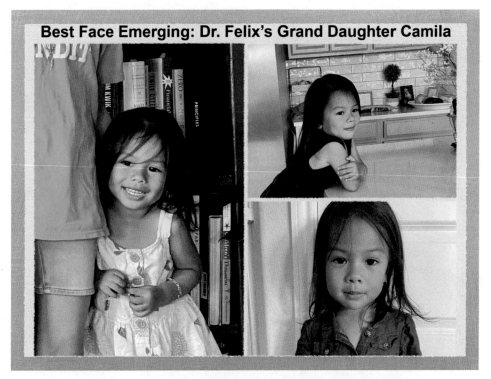

Figure 68. *No pacifier and no oral appliance so far. Just fresh home cooking by Chef Franklin each and every meal.*

Figures 68 & 69 show an update of my granddaughters Camila and her step sister SDH on their journey toward Best Face under Chef Franklin's nurture.

You do not need to be a naturopath, nor an AMD, nor a professional chef. You only need to know that your child's Best Face is founded on a fully grown maxilla. Figure 70 is an update of Mama Katie's daughters at a party.

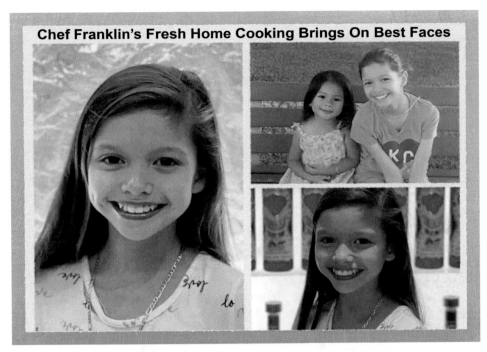

Figure 69. *These faces show what fresh home cooking based on Licensed to Thrive principles can do without oral appliances.*

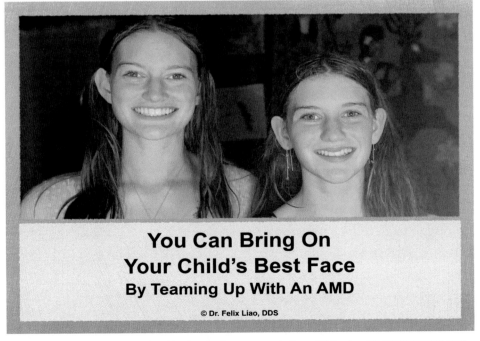

Figure 70. *From Mama Katie: "You're the first person I shared this pic with!! THANK YOU!!!!"*

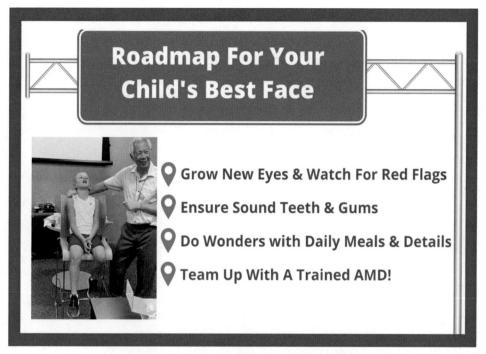

Figure 71. *The best time to evaluate and treat is ages 7–9. It's never too late, however, as long as sound healthy teeth are present.*

Final Step: Professional Support

Having read this far, your last step is finding and seeing an AMD:

- If your dentist is already trained as an AMD, you are in great hands.

- If not, you may need to nudge your dentist to get AMD Training so you can get guidance and support for your child's Best Face in your current dental office. See AMD Training in Resources on page 94.

- If neither works and you cannot wait, please see Resources on page 94 for a referral to an AMD nearest you, or an online consultation.

Your child's Best Face is now within your reach if you team up with a trained AMD to fully develop her or his maxilla.

Enjoy growing your child toward Best Face.

RESOURCES

The following is kept short intentionally to stay focused. For a more complete list of references, please see bibliographies in the recommended books below.

1. **AMD Training for Dentists:** Text/call 800-969-8035

2. **Cook2Thrive.com**[12]**:** *Thrive Your Health Through Your Kitchen for busy working professionals with Chef Franklin*

3. **Follow Case Progress:** https://bit.ly/YourChildsBestFace

4. **Referral for nearest AMD:** Email request to info@HolisticMouthSolutions.com

5. **Telemedicine consultation for a fee:** Email request to info@WholeHealthDentalCenter.com

6. **Cross-Training Summit for non-dentist healthcare professionals and AMDs to collaborate on WholeHealth:** info@HolisticMouthSolutions.com

Books by Dr. Liao on Impaired Mouth Syndrome & WholeHealth:
(Paperback readers see page 98)

1. **Six-Foot Tiger, Three-Foot Cage**[13]**:** *Take Charge of Your Health by Taking Charge of Your Mouth*

2. **Early Sirens**[14]**:** *Critical Health Warnings & Holistic Mouth Solutions for Snoring, Teeth Grinding, Jaw Clicking, Chronic Pain, Fatigue, and More*

3. **Licensed to Thrive**[15]**:** *A Mouth Owner's GPS to Vibrant Health & Innate Immunity*

4. **Relaunch Your Vitality**[16]**:** *Root Out Chronic Pain & Fatigue to Enjoy Life Again*

On Tongue-tie, Breastfeeding, Weaning, Healthier Eating, and Sleep Breathing:

1. **Academy of Orofacial Myofunctional Therapy**[17]: Its members and AMDs combine to form leading-edge expertise in physical therapy for the tongue, lips, cheek, and swallowing muscles.

2. **Breast Feeding & Breathing Competence Assessment at Birth & Treatment & Referrals**[18]

3. **Baby-Led Weaning**[19]: Gil Rapley & Tracey Murkett

4. **The Dental Diet**[20]: *The Surprising Link Between Your Teeth, Real Food, and Life-Changing Natural Health* by Dr. Steven Lin

5. **The Blood Sugar Solution**[21]: *The UltraHealthy Program for Losing Weight, Preventing Disease, and Feeling Great Now!* by Mark Hyman, MD

6. **The Weston A. Price Foundation**[22]: *Wise Traditions Diet*

7. **Nurtured Bones Newsletter**[23]: *Concise and consistently excellent tips on bone health*

8. **Sleep, Interrupted**[24]: *A physician reveals the #1 reason why so many of us are sick and tired* by Steven Y. Park, MD

9. **Sleep with Buteyko**[25]: *Stop Snoring, Sleep Apnea and Insomnia* by Patrick McKeown

CONTACT THE AUTHOR

Emails:

Dentists, Doctors, Healthcare Professionals: DrFelixLiao@gmail.com

Patients & Readers: DrFelix@HolisticMouthSolutions.com

Websites:

For healthcare professionals: www.HolisticMouthSolutions.com

For patients seeking consultation: www.WholeHealthDentalCenter.com

Facebook:

For healthcare professionals: www.facebook.com/HolisticMouthSolutions

For patients seeking consultation: www.facebook.com/wholehealthdentalcenter

Instagram:

www.instagram.com/6_foot_tiger

LinkedIn:

www.linkedin.com/company/HolisticMouthSolutions

REFERENCES

1. **Syndrome (Lexico):** https://www.lexico.com/en/definition/syndrome

2. **Dr. Takashi Ono:** https://www.froggymouth.com/e2/en/concept

3. **Dr. Joel Fuhrman MD:** https://www.theepochtimes.com/cytokine-storm-when-the-immune-system-goes-awry_4271020.html?utm_source=healthnoe&utm_campaign=health-2022-02-11&utm_medium=email&est=0tAlLMSTqzHIPqH7eUI7bT1UcfqqEKz96mbL1ZwFQcXm+9z3Zuiu4hT+HXqE

4. **CDC:** https://www.cdc.gov/genomics/disease/epigenetics.htm

5. **Fetal head circumference:** https://jamanetwork.com/journals/jamapediatrics/article-abstract/2757542

6. **PCBs:** https://oceanservice.noaa.gov/facts/pcbs.html

7. **Organo-chlorine pesticides:** https://www.ncbi.nlm.nih.gov/pmc/articles/PMC5464684

8. **2004 EWG study:** https://www.ewg.org/research/body-burden-pollution-newborns

9. **2015 report:** https://pubmed.ncbi.nlm.nih.gov/26433469

10. **EWG in 2018:** https://www.ewg.org/news-insights/news-release/2018/10/roundup-breakfast-part-2-new-tests-weed-killer-found-all-kids

11. **US Geological Survey:** https://www.usgs.gov/special-topics/water-science-school/science/pharmaceuticals-water

12. **Cook2Thrive.com:** https://www.cook2thrive.com

13. **Six-Foot Tiger, Three-Foot Cage:** https://www.amazon.com/Six-Foot-Tiger-Three-Foot-Cage-Charge/dp/1944177590

14. **Early Sirens:** https://www.amazon.com/Early-Sirens-Critical-Warnings-Solutions-ebook/dp/B0762S8G9B

15. **Licensed to Thrive:** https://www.amazon.com/Licensed-Thrive-Owners-Vibrant-Immunity-ebook/dp/B08R93GNB4/ref=sr_1_1?crid=2RS4XK6VJGFWN&keywords=licensed+to+thrive+book&qid=1641055620&s=books&sprefix=licensed+to+thrive+book,stripbooks,89&sr=1-1

16. **Relaunch Your Vitality:** https://holisticmouthsolutions.com/relaunch-your-vitality

17. **Academy of Orofacial Myofunctional Therapy:** https://www.aomtinfo.org

18. **Breast Feeding & Breathing Competence Assessment At Birth & Treatment & Referrals:** https://www.littlesproutspeech.com

19. **Baby Led Weaning:** https://www.amazon.com/Baby-Led-Weaning-Completely-Expanded-Anniversary-ebook/dp/B07H3GS91K/ref=sr_1_5?crid=2MMY8SBQL94C&keywords=baby+led+weaning&qid=1641055451&s=books&sprefix=baby+led+we%2Cstripbooks%2C89&sr=1-5

20. **The Dental Diet:** https://www.amazon.com/Dental-Diet-Surprising-between-Life-Changing/dp/1401953190/ref=tmm_pap_swatch_0?_encoding=UTF8&qid=&sr=

21. **The Blood Sugar Solution:** https://www.amazon.com/Blood-Sugar-Solution-UltraHealthy-Preventing-ebook/dp/B004QX07AK/ref=sr_1_9?keywords=Mark+Hyman&qid=1641056868&s=books&sr=1-9

22. **The Weston A. Price Foundation:** https://www.westonaprice.org

23. **Nurtured Bones Newsletter:** https://www.nurturedbones.com

24. **Sleep, Interrupted:** https://www.amazon.com/Sleep-Interrupted-Steven-Park-M-D-ebook/dp/B002R5B2GM

25. **Sleep with Buteyko:** https://www.amazon.com/Sleep-Buteyko-Insomnia-Suitable-Children-ebook/dp/B08L3S85V3/ref=sr_1_3?crid=2UZVE22MQXDIH&keywords=patrick+mckeown+books&qid=1641639276&s=digital-text&sprefix=Patrick+Mck,digital-text,91&sr=1-3